U0276968

守在生命的边缘

医者沉思录

主 编 毛一雷

中国协和医科大学出版社

北 京

图书在版编目（CIP）数据

守在生命的边缘：医者沉思录 / 毛一雷主编. -- 北京：中国协和医科大学出版社, 2024.9. -- ISBN 978-7-5679-2467-3

Ⅰ. R199.2

中国国家版本馆CIP数据核字第2024J77R73号

主　　编　毛一雷
责任编辑　李元君　　白　兰
封面设计　邱晓俐
责任校对　张　麓
责任印制　黄艳霞
出版发行　**中国协和医科大学出版社**
　　　　　（北京市东城区东单三条9号　邮编100730　电话010-65260431）
网　　址　www.pumcp.com
印　　刷　三河市龙大印装有限公司
开　　本　880mm×1230mm　　1/32
印　　张　11.125
字　　数　300千字
版　　次　2024年9月第1版
印　　次　2024年9月第1次印刷
定　　价　78.00元

编者名单

主　　编　毛一雷

副 主 编　汪道远　杨华瑜　刘燕华　郑思华
　　　　　　　孙铭浩

文章作者　（按姓氏笔画排序）

于丽华　王子怡　王禹歆　仇毓东
白雪莉　丛亚丽　邢宝才　吕文良
伊保康　刘　辰　刘　明　刘允怡
花苏榕　杜顺达　杨　田　吴麟杰
沈　峰　张　戈　张群华　陈　伟
陈亚进　陈进宏　周　杰　周伟平
周军彬　郎婧婧　钦伦秀　袁声贤
耿小平　徐　达　徐　骁　曹　君
彭吉润　傅麒宁

序　一

当毛一雷教授把他的新书《守在生命的边缘——医者沉思录》的样稿交到我手上并邀请我为之作序时，我深感荣幸之余，又感叹于毛教授的精力旺盛。这是我第二次给他的书写序了。很少有医生能像他这样，在出色地完成繁重的医教研工作之余，还能有如此丰富的人生、广阔的社交和勤奋的创作。

我和毛教授的缘分起始于1999年，那年他被北京协和医院作为引进人才招揽到外科，在此之前他曾在北欧最著名的瑞典隆德大学（Lund University）获得外科博士学位，又在美国哈佛大学完成博士后训练，同时在美国麻省总医院（MGH）肿瘤外科完成临床培训。2002年，协和医院在原有基础外科肝脏外科专业组的基础之上，成立了独立的肝脏外科中心，毛教授就是在彼时加入了肝脏外科，从此我与他的交往更为紧密。当时，我仍每天在病房查房，也经常进手术室做手术，算得上是毛教授的老师，随着交往日久，竟然成了忘年交。

在我眼中，毛教授不仅仅是个优秀且全面的外科医生，他在面对协和医院繁重的临床、教学、科研工作对医生提出的近乎苛刻的要求时，也总是游刃有余，在自己的专业领域表现得极其出色，他三次被评为北京协和医院"十大最佳外科教授"，足见他的实力得到广泛认可；同时，他又是个不走寻常路的人，他参加了南极冰盖最高点昆仑科考站的初建，曾两次自驾进藏，在珠峰大本营看过日照金山，在阿拉斯加的冰河驾舟漂流，也在非洲马赛马拉的稀树大草原上追逐过动物大迁徙，在尼罗鳄出没的尼罗河划过船，在爱琴海博斯普鲁斯海峡边跑步……有时险象环生，也经历过生死考验，每每听他讲述这些神奇的经历，都会使老朽感受到些许年轻人的激荡胸怀。

当然，他还是一个笔耕不辍的作者、作家，除了撰写了很多高水平的专业论文、著作之外，他还把他的南极经历以日记的形式写成《生命印记——南极之巅》一书（也是邀请我作的序），后来它的英文版 *The Top of The Bottom of The World* 在美国又得以出版。他更是创办了一本高质量的SCI外科期刊——*Hepatobillary Surgery and Nutrition*（*HBSN*），并将其发展成为世界著名的外科期刊。

虽然我年事已高，但阅读还没有成为负担，经年累月的学习习惯还是使得我读文章有享受感。本书所集结的文章我大多都读过，毕竟毛教授的 *HBSN* 是肝胆外科专业领域少有的中国人创办的高质量国际性期刊。2020年4月起，这确实是一种有益的尝试，我对此非常赞赏。虽然不少国外期刊也有类似的专栏，但国内创办的期刊确实鲜有这方面的探索。医学人文和伦理是医学中不可或缺的一部分，是医学的初心和起源，也是医学的温度和尺度。*HBSN* 的这一专栏在过去的几年里，陆续发表了一系列广大医疗工作者、人民群众、社会和政府所关心和聚焦的医学人文、医学伦理和医疗政策相关问题，为不同观点的争鸣和讨论提供了一个畅所欲言的平台，为医疗管理者在政策制定、规则优化方面提供了参考，为国际社会了解中国真实的医疗环境、医疗政策打开了一扇窗。

本书好几篇文章从不同角度就新技术的开展和普及在伦理、管理等方面的影响展开了讨论，在我看来是非常有必要的。医学进步需要创新，且实践是检验真理的唯一标准，但在实践过程中，总难以避免地付出一定代价。如何更科学、更安全地推进新技术的应用，考验的是医生医疗水平和成长欲望之间的平衡，更考验医疗安全管理水平，相信每个读者都会有各自不同的观点和见解。本书所涉及的话题都有与此类似的特点：重要，却没有一致或简单的答案。相信这些文章不仅是医生们感兴趣的，也会是大众读者很感兴趣的。

　　本书虽然是遴选很多位医学、医政专家的文章并汇总而成，但文章通俗易懂，把这几十篇文字风格不同、话题不同的探讨集合成一本书，非但不显杂乱，反而相得益彰。本书话题都是由毛教授拟定并约稿的，每篇文章之前都有他亲笔所写的导读，读者从中可以更深入地了解医生的所思所想、所忧所虑，也可以更加理解医疗政策背后的底层逻辑。当然，每个人对问题都会有自己的解读和思考，这本书可以起到抛砖引玉的作用，为读者带来更多的思考空间。

　　岁月就像手术室里的时钟，在还来不及感到疲惫的时候就匆匆而过，一晃几十年，当年的"毛头小伙子"如今也已经成长为著名的外科专家、学者、导师了。我在耄耋之年回首过往种种，还是要庆幸能和毛教授这位同行有这段忘年交。都说严肃的医生千篇一律，有趣的灵魂万中无一，而毛一雷正是那有着有趣灵魂的严肃外科医生，相信他的新书一定能够为读者带来别致的阅读体验和思考。

钟守先

2024 年 5 月

于东单北极阁三条

序 二

医界的一线感言实属难能可贵

毛一雷教授请我为医生们编写的这本书作个序，有点诚惶诚恐，因我一向是患者或是代亲友同事求医的角色，对医生群体推崇有加，对于医道之事不敢一本正经地胡说八道。我对医生群体的兴趣也由来已久，当从社会学角度研究中产阶级时，医生群体和律师群体是欧美中产阶级研究中最典型的群体。说到中产，往往意味着专业技能、专业标准、专业保障与专业伦理，本书与医生的专业伦理关联颇多，所触及的话题也是社会所高度关注的，不少知识点弥补了我的认知空白。本书在漫谈形式下的文风颇有通俗、举重若轻的特点，所以先睹为快之余说点感想倒是未尝不可。

如果我站在一名用心而又不那么情绪化的患者的角度，去阅读医生们撰写的这些文章时，的确会与医生们的视角有些区别。我曾如此建议一位即将上岗的学医小辈：面对患者要尽量随和友好，并且尽可能多地给他们普及些健康知识。后来，他与我谈他的一些前辈们的想法：你们只要能坚持认真看病就不错了，因为没有时间和精力去表达友好。对此说法我始终持保留意见。2018年我在上海同济医院住院，施宝民医生是我的主治医生。住院期间，施大夫在查房时除了帮我分析健康状况，还会为我讲解一些健康知识，从胃酸、胆汁，到B超和"胰腺炎人格"。当时我意识到原来真有医生能做到对患者友善，帮患者普及医学知识，可见医患关系的模式还是有很多探讨、探索的空间的。尤其是现在创建了更完善的就医机制，实现了从预约挂号、有序排队候诊、电子病历与开单检查、医患交谈与问询，到处方开具与取药、实施手术与住院办理的全触点服务流程。我们需要考虑在该流程中如何很好地平衡就医效率和服务质量、患者感受和医者诊断以及患者福利和医护利益等之间的关系。站在全面维护患者福利的角度，还应该将患者在院诊疗之后的服务机制纳入考虑——居家预后的社区卫生服务追踪、术后或后续治疗照护的专项服务、临终关怀服务的建设等。

我们寄希望于技术进步为医疗服务与健康管理带来更大的助益，如互联网医院、智能读图与诊断、新药物和新手术技术的应用，都赋能医者亦助益患者。本书中关于腹腔镜手术技术的应用有比较多的讨论，与所通常看到的外行对于技术的推崇不同，作者们不仅严肃地讨论了腹腔镜的应用价值及其带给患者的实际利益，而且从患者获益最大化角度提出了："即使是先进新技术，也要充分考虑不能带给患者足够利益的'有所不为'的场景。"

在公共卫生意义上有很多课题值得重视，本书提到的医保费用计量的DRG方法对我这个外行来说是冷知识。考虑到中国医保网覆盖面建设的有限时长，当前所取得的成效值得称道，且DRG中国方案的试点推行对于优化中国医保体系的可支撑性很有意义。本书提到的基层医疗困境话题，也非常有意义。身边那些在基层医院诊治无效后再转至北京、上海等大城市就医的亲朋好友的经历，使我切身感受到基层医疗资源的有限性和诊疗质量存在的问题。在现有改革举措下这些问题尚未得到根本改善，更何谈在基层医院，诸如脑功能康复、罕见病治疗、梅尼埃病患者照料这些问题，困难就更大了。关于新一代医护人才培养，这是从三甲医院到基层医院普遍存在的问题。尽管本书有文专门讲的是住院医生规范化培训，但目前在医学生群体中所出现的主动首选临床医学专业的人少，学习时缺少专业方向感和专业爱好，学习后缺乏从医的理想和热情，从医时的培训辅导带领机制滞后的现象……不仅仅反映出当前高等教育与社会职业实践前沿联通不足的通病，而且也说明急需从医疗实践、技术变迁、病患发展以及原有教学模式滞后的现状中，全面反思并重构医护人才培养及其能力提升强化机制。书中有文专门介绍了医护人员的饮食健康现状，即医院人力资源管理中专业群体的健康管理问题，这也会牵制医学生们对未来职业的展望。书中有文从女医生的角度讨论性别在医疗资源中的特色本身也是个有价值的视角。

我读完本书后的第一反应，就是应当发挥本人所在数据分析机构零点有数的专业作用——不同类型患者的医疗人类学经历叙述、患者医疗服务全触点体验评价、疾病场景中患者的感受转化和行为变化的追踪研究、医患在医疗过程中的互动关系与医患诉求平衡性研究、医生从业感受的长期追踪研究。我所在机构参与的医疗研究涵盖了中国糖尿病患者人类学研究，个人疼痛史研究，艾滋病与性传播疾病的长期追踪研究，多类OTC药物接受度研究，多类慢性病追踪研究，包括传染性非典型肺炎（SARS）、禽流感、甲型H1N1流感和新冠病毒感染在内的多类传染病的公共传播特点与社会影响研究，以及社区医疗服务模式的对比分析等。我深切地感受到，具有不同诊疗专业和特长的医护群体，如果能够更合理地与具有研究分析特长的专业群体合作，那么在科研方面就会取得较预期更好的成果。比如医者出身的医院管理群体与后勤管理群体、技术管理群体以及服务设计群体展开高质量的合作，可推动医疗机构的综合能力有所突破。

为毛一雷教授主编的《守在生命的边缘——医者沉思录》一书所撰序言于此奉上。愿各位读者于阅读之中有所感、有所得。

——零点有数董事长袁岳

北京大学社会学博士

哈佛大学公共管理硕士

前　言

屈指算来，本人从医已三十余载，做过很多手术，写过很多论文，也做过很多科研，还创刊了一本专业杂志（*Hepatobiliary Surgery and Nutrition*，*HBSN*），但内心深处始终感觉还应该再多做些什么。

作为一门需要温度的学科，医学所关注的绝不应该仅局限于其"科学"属性，更应该包括其"人文"属性。医学中的许多问题是医生、患者、社会和政府都应当共同关注的，因为这些问题不仅涉及人性和道德、健康和科学、利益和资源，也与政策和管理、公平和稳定密切相关。而即便是我这样"资深"的医疗工作者，对于这些问题也存在很多认知不足、思辨不清之处，更有不少如鲠在喉却又无处倾诉的苦恼，而且工作中接触过的很多同行专家学者，都与我一样有类似的感慨。

因此，从2020年4月起，我决定在自己创刊的*HBSN*杂志上开设医学伦理－人文专栏，初衷就是想提供一个小小的平台，就医疗领域的一些热点、焦点问题，邀请国内相应领域的专家、学者撰稿，深入分析，自由阐述，使其充分表达个人观点。对于绝大多数人而言，医学专业杂志都是冰冷、艰涩、玄奥的，尤其以循证为基础的医学专业文章通常充斥着一串串冰冷的数字、艰涩难懂的统计学方法，以及各种玄奥的假设和理论。而这个小小的专栏，即便是普通读者也能轻松阅读。

在过去的三年多里，*HBSN*每期都会拟定一个主题，内容涉及医疗新技术的应用和推广、医生的培养和成长、医疗决策、临床科研、医患关系、临终关怀、院外医疗、医保政策、DRG支付政策等一系列医疗领域的热点和焦点问题。这些问题都存在不同程度的争议，没有所谓的标准答案，但每篇文章都由相关领域卓有建树的学者撰文，来自每一位作者多年的专业经验和严肃思考。这些文章呈现出一种集活泼生动与理性、深刻务实于一体的思考文风，不仅令人耳目一新，又极具启发性。后来这些文章又在网络上的丁香园平台登载，进一步扩大了受众面，从而引发了更广泛的关注和理性讨论。这在当今喧嚣浮躁的互联网时代是难能可贵的，也正是我希望看到的——自由、理性、包容、热烈的思想展露和交流有助于认知的提升和社会的进步。

然而，上述文章在时间和空间上如此分散，互联网的记忆又是如此短暂，这让我深感不安和遗憾。不安是因为这些文章都是作者们思想的结晶，不容辜负；遗憾是因为时代的话题层出不穷，真金也容易被掩埋。我总觉得还需要再多做些什么，所以我萌发了一种强烈的想法，要把这些分散的文章集结成书，让它们以另一种形式整体"重生"，而且书名我也想好了，就叫《守在生命的边缘——医者沉思录》吧。

医生这一职业，常常与生死打交道，"守在生命的边缘"，一线隔阴阳，一念分神魔。有成功，也有失败，有人性的光辉，也有人类的孱弱。一个"守"字，一方面是表达在疾病面前，医生往往处在被动防守一方；另一方面表达了医生这一职业要求包含"守卫""守护"的内容，是与患者共同面对、抵抗疾病的战友；再一方面，也有积极对抗疾病的意义在内，所谓"进攻是最好的防守"，医学的不断探索和进步正是"以攻为守"的最佳诠释。书名的副标题是"医者沉思录"，灵感来自哲学著作《沉思录》，其作者古罗马皇帝马可·奥勒留（Marcus Aurelius，公元121—180）被誉为世界历史上唯一一位"帝王哲学家"，是西方斯多葛派代表人物之一，其思想显露出早期辩证唯物主义的端倪，认为只有物质形式的事物才是真实的存在，辩证法和修辞学是两大思考工具，强调理性思维的作用。他在伦理学方面则提出了最早的"个人主义"和"平等"观念，认为个人修养要有四类美德：智慧，所以辨别善恶；公道，以便应付悉合分际；勇敢，借以终止苦痛；节制，不为物欲所役。这些思想在很大程度上都契合医生这一行业。医生，是最容易从日常工作中引发对人生、职业、社会、宇宙、哲学等问题深思的一群人，他们的工作不只是治病救人，也是一场自我修行，他们对人性的洞察、生命的敬畏、科学的探索、社会的理解乃至哲学的思考，可能会给更多人带来不一样的启发。

我去过不少地方，足迹几乎遍布世界，从喧嚣拥挤的摩登都市到人迹罕至的荒原戈壁，从万物生长的热带雨林到寸草不生的极地冰原，从风情迥异的异国他乡到江山辽阔的祖国家园，见识过多元的文化思维、迥异的风俗习惯、奇妙的动物植物、壮美的山河湖海，我深感多元化的视角、观点对于一颗健康美好的灵魂的重要性丝毫不亚于营养均衡的食物对于健全、健康的身体的重要性。当读者朋友们在闲暇之余，捧起这本翰墨芬芳的书，希望你们能感受到来自思考的力量和裨益，也希望本书能为你们带来更深刻、更有益的思索。

最后，我要感谢我多年的好友，零点有数集团的袁岳先生，他也是北京哈佛校友会理事，感谢他在繁忙的工作之余抽出时间为本书作序；更要感谢我尊敬的老师，北京协和医院外科专家钟守先先生，感谢他在耄耋之年仍愿为我的新书作序，更感谢他多年来对我的无私支持和帮助。

毛一雷

2024 年 5 月

于北京东单三条

目　录

让公众走近了解医疗从业者

让医患相关热点回暖

医疗技术何以选择，不负患者？

杏林深深自沉思

让医疗步入公众视野

让**公众**
走近了解
医疗 从业者

主编导读（一）

每天劝患者合理膳食的医生们，自己好好吃饭了吗？

国人的三餐到底怎么吃才算对？医务人员的膳食结构作出表率了吗？

近年来，对于国人膳食结构的合理调配是大家最为关心的，也是最具争议的话题。一方面由于生活水平的提高，日常饮食中能量和脂类的摄入明显增加，社会上悄然增加了众多的需要减肥的人群，有人把减肥当成终身努力的目标。民众之中尤其是女性同胞们热议并坚持着各种各样减重方式，新的方法也层出不穷，其中包括节食、运动、生酮饮食、时间限制性进食等，各有各的理论，莫衷一是，无标准可循。另一方面在中国的传统医学文化的长期熏陶下，很多民众自己经常扮演着"半个医生"的角色（不像西方文化里，要么是医生，要么不是医生那么清晰）。

我们常常能够观察到中年人群尤其是七大姑八大姨们，基于多年的生活经验，他们自然而然地变成医生了，如对于手术前后的患者会有凌驾于医嘱之上的执着的指导原则：油腻要忌口、辛辣要忌口、海鲜要忌口等。对于日常生活中如何避免体重超重，如何维持健康生活状态，更是有执着的信念。但事实是，发福的人群、有富贵病的人群没有因此而减少。

最近我国颁布了新版的公众食品指南，几乎同时美国也新颁布了有关饮食指南。为了解除大家包括我个人的困惑，提供一个相对权威、正确的饮食方式，*HBSN*主编专程采访了北京协和医院临床营养科主任陈伟教授。陈教授在参考了中美两国新版的饮食指南后，把相关内容写成了一篇综述文章并公开发表。

在文章中，除了公众饮食结构以外，陈教授还对于我国的医务工作者在饮食情况进行了调查统计，结果发现虽然身为医务工作者，但实际上在饮食方面并没有起到表率作用。

谁来守护医务人员的饮食健康?

陈　伟

北京协和医院　临床营养科

合理膳食、适量运动、心理平衡、戒烟限酒是世界卫生组织提出守护健康的四大基石，在此强调合理营养在健康守护中发挥最重要的基础性作用。大量流行病学证据表明，健康的饮食习惯不仅可以满足营养素需求、保持机体健康，还可以降低营养相关的慢性非传染性疾病的发生风险。

工作忙，总吃外卖

由于医务人员长期居于一线承担繁重的医疗任务，紧张的就业环境与不规律的用餐和作息使得医务工作者的心理和生理都承担了巨大压力，使得本应是带头践行健康生活方式和行为的一类健康引导群体，反而成了最不注重自身健康生活方式的一类人群。

就最近美团外卖发布的《2020中国医生群体饮食报告》来看，仅2020年上半年，全国有700多万名医生叫外卖，订单总量超过1.7亿单。因此，医务人员的膳食营养乃至健康状态都是一个值得关注的问题。

有研究发现，急诊、ICU病房的医务人员有不良饮食习惯的比例更高，其中早餐的保证率只有67%，谷物、水果和奶制品的摄入均不足，而畜禽肉摄入则过量，表现出比一般人群更为严重的膳食营养问题。

一项关于医生饮食的调研

为调查我国医务人员实际生活中的饮食营养摄入、生活方式及对健康的影响，并进一步寻找有效提高医务人员的营养健康水平的科学依据，中国营养学会临床营养分会于2020年6月推出了线上营养自测调研系统，在网络平台展开征集活动。

本次调研主要针对全国31个省、自治区、直辖市不同等级的医院，涵盖多科室医务人员，从日常生活情况、健康行为、食物及营养素摄入情况、健康感知及疾病情况等方面进行调研，共收集了9196份有效问卷，回收率高达95.6%。

本次调研从三个维度包括食物摄入和营养状况、行为与生活习惯情况、日常健康状况等进行分析，并侧重不同性别、不同科室的调查，探讨影响医务人员营养素摄入和健康状况的相关因素。

结果显示，参与调查人员中内科（20%）、营养科（19%）、妇产科（18%）、外科（12%）医务人员的不良饮食及生活行为发生率较高，原因如下：①整体工作繁忙且工作时间长（每周工作时长超40小时者高达80.51%），每天很难保持良好的睡眠质量和睡眠时长（少于7小时/天者占74.78%）。②由于工作繁忙，在家进餐时间较少（在家进餐＜7次/周的比例达33.31%）、不能按时用餐（30.46%）且用餐时间短（进餐时长＜10分钟者占34.65%）。③日常运动少（运动时间少于40分钟/天者占73.74%），多数无固定日晒且长时间久坐（久坐时间超过2小时/天者占68.07%），对身体健康造成不良影响，有32%的医务人员有超重甚至肥胖的问题。

①健康状况方面，常见易发疾病的患病情况从高到低分别为视力下降或疲劳（81.32%）、感冒（62.20%）、慢性胃肠炎（33.05%）、便秘（31.94%）及经常性口角炎/溃疡（13.80%）。②常见已知慢性病患病情况从高到低分别为血脂异常（21.50%）、心血管疾病（8.42%）、肿瘤（5.87%）和糖尿病（2.49%）。糖尿病、心血管疾病、血脂异常的患病率方面，女性医生低于男性医生（$P < 0.05$），但女性医生恶性肿瘤的患病率高于男性医生（$P < 0.05$）。

此外，我们以《中国居民膳食指南》（2016版）中提供的健康人推荐营养素摄入量为参考值，发现超50%医务工作者每日膳食摄入量不达标：59.65%医务工作者每日谷类摄入不足250g，63.41%医务工作者每日蔬菜摄入不足450g，58.88%医务工作者每日水果摄入不足300g，而有70.2%医务人员每日大豆摄入超过10g；41.81%医务工作者每日坚果摄入不足10g，65.95%医务工作者每日乳制品摄入不足300g，但36.54%医务人员每日禽畜肉类的摄入超过100g；每日水产品的摄入不足100g的医务工作者占88.75%。

分析营养素摄入量汇总结果发现，参加调查的医务人员的总能量摄入偏低，且三大产热营养素所提供热能的比例不合理，碳水化合物占比过低（46.67%）、脂肪占比过高（35.37%）；除蛋白质、铁和烟酸摄入充足外，多种营养素摄入不足，其中对维生素A、维生素C、锌、硒四类营养成分的摄入量远远低于推荐营养素摄入量。

综合分析医务人员营养成分摄入不足的影响因素发现，这与其饮食行为密切相关。其中，在家用餐次数少（每周少于7次）、用餐时间不规律、进餐用时短（少于30分钟）的医务人员中各种营养素摄入不足率高于在家用餐次数多、用餐规律、进食时间长的；而自带工作餐者的维生素A、维生素B_2、钙、钾摄入不足率低于食堂或外出就餐者（$P < 0.05$）。

医生的饮食健康状况不佳

通过本次截面调研结果，我们发现中国医务人员的不良饮食及健康状况不容乐观，虽然在问卷中医务人员的健康知识水平较高并且存在通过饮食生活获得健康的意愿，但是付诸健康行动的能力却远远不足。

医务人员普遍工作强度大，无法全身心投入自身健康管理，只有让营养干预以制度的形式，进入日常生活。比如国家卫生健康委2020年推出健康食堂的工作，要求医疗机构的职工食堂达到健康食堂的标准，才能在日常生活中守护医务人员的健康，再进一步从健康自身到引领全国人民的健康未来。

从医院管理角度来说，关注医务人员自身的生活质量和心理状况，改善医务人员的工作状态、改善医院食堂的营养和口味，减少医务人员外食的机会，都有助于提高其健康状况。而对于医务人员来说，也应该增强自身饮食和健康意识，清醒地了解健康获得是靠同样的努力才能得到的。

2021年5月发布的《中国居民膳食指南》（2021版）中进一步提出科学营养，按量吃饭的要求，将居民膳食与健康紧密结合在一起。总之，医生群体作为高文化知识、高科学素养的群体，更应该重视改善营养与健康层面的保护，在健康中国发挥引领作用。

参考文献

［1］Report on Chinese Residents' Chronic Diseases and Nutrition (2020). Chinese State Council. December 23, 2020. Available online: http://www.gov.cn/xinwen/2020-12/24/content_5572983.htm

［2］Healthy China (2019－2030). Healthy China Action Promotion Committee. July 9, 2019. Available online: http://www.gov.cn/xinwen/2019-07/15/content_5409694. htm

［3］Chinese Doctor Diet Report. Meituan. August 18, 2020. Available online: https://ishare.ifeng.com/c/s/v002tGQzZjf9e9Shg6-_fxIMOwzQeOS8yIOYqg27--4MXZ78I

［4］Zhu XR. Investigation on Dietary Habits and Nutrition Intake of Emergency ICU Medical Staffs. World Latest Med 2018; 18: 11-2.

［5］The Writing Committee of the Report on Cardiovascular Health and Diseases in China. Interpretation of Report on Cardiovascular Health and Diseases in China 2019. Chin J Cardiovasc Med 2020; 35: 833-54.

［6］Scientific Research Report on Dietary Guidelines for Chinese (2021). Chinese Nutrition Society 2020. Available online: https://www.cnsoc.org/learnnews/422120203.html

［7］U.S. Department of Agriculture and U.S. Department of Health and Human Services. Dietary Guidelines for Americans, 2020－2025. 9th Edition. December 2020. Available online: https://www.dietaryguidelines.gov/sites/default/files/2020-12/Dietary_Guidelines_for_ Americans_2020-2025.pdf

［8］Chinese Nutrition Society. Chinese Dietary Guidelines (2016). Beijing: People's Medical Publishing House, 2016: 115-6.

Dietary health of medical workers: who's taking care of it?

Chen Wei

Department of Clinical Nutrition, Peking Union Medical College Hospital, PUMC, Chinese Academy of Medical Sciences, Beijing, China

The World Health Organization has suggested that people should follow these four rules of maintaining healthy eating habits, a tobacco-free lifestyle, regular physical activities, and an environment for social and emotional well-being, all of which constitutes a healthy lifestyle. Among them, a healthy diet plays the most important role. It has been well-established that healthy eating habits not only meet one's nutritional needs, but also lower one's risk of having nutrition-related chronic non-communicable diseases.

According to the *"Report on Chinese Residents' Chronic Diseases and Nutrition"* issued by the State Council in December 2020 [1], the chronic diseases were the leading causes of national mortality, accounting for 88.5% of the total deaths in China in 2019. Herein, the cerebrovascular diseases, cancer and chronic respiratory diseases were related to lethality, altogether accounting for 80.7% of the total mortality. What's worse, there is a tendency towards an increase in the prevalence of such chronic diseases in the Chinese people in the next few decades, mainly because of two reasons. For one thing, many Chinese people still live an unhealthy life for their imbalanced diet with excessive consumption of fat, oil, sodium, and insufficient intake of fruits, beans, and dairy products. For another thing, the rising incidence of obesity in China directly leads to increased prevalence of the chronic diseases, too. It has been showed that the rate of overweight or obesity was over 50% in adults, 19% in children under 6 and 10.4% in children or adolescents aged 6-17, respectively. In correspondence with the rise in obesity/overweight incidence, there is an increased prevalence of hypertension, diabetes, hypercholesterolemia, chronic obstructive pulmonary disease, and cancer in 2019, higher than those in 2015. To tackle with these serious issues, the "Healthy China 2030" initiative has set a comprehensive strategic plan, with implementation of crucial health-and-nutrition-related policy, including health knowledge popularization, promotion of a balanced diet as well as prevention and control of major chronic diseases [2].

Healthcare workers play a key role in practicing the "Healthy China 2030" initiative and reducing the burden of chronic diseases. However, due to the heavy workloads, stressful working environment, and irregular work schedules, many healthcare workers often sacrificed their own physical and emotional needs, in an effort to provide care for the patients. Meituan (food delivery company) has released the "Chinese Doctor Diet Report 2020", which showed that more than 7 million doctors have placed over 170 million orders for take-out foods in China, just in the first half of 2020 [3]. Except for eating junk foods instead of swapping for a healthy diet, some other unhealthy behaviors also have impact on people's health, such as skipping breakfast, lacking cereals, fruits, and dairy products in the meals, and consuming too much meat and poultry. Among doctors with various background, those working in the emergency room and ICU wards had a greater tendency of being afflicted by an unhealthy diet [4].

The improper diet structure is closely correlated with the risk of developing chronic diseases. The "China Cardiovascular Health and Disease Report 2019" [5] pointed out that cardiovascular disease was ranked as the leading cause of death; however, 2/3 of major coronary events and 2/5 of acute ischemic stroke could be prevented through

守在生命的边缘
医者沉思录

adherence to healthy lifestyle. Through a risk attribution analysis, the 2010－2012 Chinese Nutrition and Health Survey found that [6] most cases of cardiovascular death were attributed to excessive sodium intake (＞2.0g/d) (17.3%), identified as the main contributing factor. Besides, the cases were also attributed to low fruits intake (＜300.0g/d) (11.5%), low omega-3 fatty acids intake (＜250.0mg/d) (9.7%), low nuts ingestion (＜250.0mg/d) (8.2%), whole grains deficiency (＜125.0g/d) (8.1%) and low consumption of vegetables (＜400.0g/d) (7.3%). From 1982 to 2012, there was a transition in the diet structure of Chinese people towards reduction in grains (especially coarse grains), fresh vegetables, fruits (fewer than 50g of fruits daily per person) and increased intake in animal foods and oil. A trend of reduction in salts and soy sauce ingestion was observed, though the average sodium intake is still as high as 10.5g daily per person. Therefore, to improve the prevention and management of chronic diseases, there is a necessity to establish health policy which aims at government, society, and individuals, with practice of promoting the health service, enhancing nutritional education and boosting people's well-being in all aspects.

Western developed countries also face similar dilemma. The majority of the American population did not meet recommendations of the Dietary Guidelines for their usual dietary intake, which might be associated with the rising incidence of nutrition-related chronic diseases. The U.S. Department of Agriculture (USDA) and the Health and Human Services (HHS) update the dietary guidelines every 5 years to attempt to improve people's eating habits. The most recent guideline (2020 to 2025) provided four major principles to help people maintain health and prevent chronic diseases throughout their entire life [7]: (I) following a healthy dietary habit; (II) choosing the nutrient-rich foods; (III) achieving a balanced diet comprising all kinds of food groups and limiting high-calorie foods; (IV) restricting alcohol and foods rich in added sugar, saturated fat and salt.

In order to investigate the impact of different dietary patterns on the health status of healthcare workers and find scientific evidence to effectively improve their health condition, the Clinical Nutrition Branch of the Chinese Nutrition Society conducted an online nutrition survey to measure healthcare workers' nutritional status, lifestyle, and health condition in 31 provinces, cities and municipalities in China in June 2020. In the survey, selected healthcare workers were enquired about their lifestyle, health behavior, food and nutrient intake, disease status, perception, and knowledge on health maintenance, etc. A total of 9,196 valid questionnaires were collected, with a response rate of 95.6%. The data were analyzed from three perspectives (food intake and nutritional status, behaviors and health condition) and the respondents' gender and working departments were taken as stratifiers for subsequent analysis. The results showed that workers from departments of internal medicine (20%), nutrition (19%), obstetrics and gynecology (18%) and surgery (12%) had more chances of having an unhealthy diet and lifestyle than those from other medical departments. The extended and busy work shifts (80.51% of them worked $\geqslant$ 40hours/week), irregular sleep pattern with poor sleeping quality (74.78% slept $\leqslant$ 7hours/day), limited access to home-cooked foods (33.31% of them ate at home for $<$ 7times/week), irregular eating behavior (30.46%), short mealtime (34.65% $<$ 10minutes per meal), a sedentary lifestyle with daily exercise deficiency (73.74% of them exercised for $\leqslant$ 40minutes/day), lack of sunlight exposure (68.07% kept sitting for longer than 2hours/day). All these behaviors had unfavorable impact on the health condition, with development of overweight or obesity in 32% of the healthcare workers who were investigated. Other common complaints included blurred vision or fatigue (81.32%), being apt to catch cold (62.20%), chronic gastroenteritis (33.05%), constipation (31.94%), and recurrent canker sores (13.80%). The frequently reported chronic diseases comprised dyslipidemia (21.50%), cardiovascular diseases (8.42%), cancer

守在生命的边缘
医者沉思录

(5.87%), and diabetes (2.49%). Compared to the male doctors, the females had a lower rate of diabetes, cardiovascular diseases, dyslipidemia, but a higher rate of cancer (all $P < 0.05$).

Additionally, we found that more than 50% of healthcare workers did not meet the daily nutrient intake allowance recommended by the "Chinese Dietary Guidelines (2016)" [8], with grain intake $< 250g/day$ in 59.65% of subjects, vegetable intake $< 450g/day$ in 63.41%, fruit intake $< 300g/day$ in 58.88%, bean intake $< 10g/day$ in 70.2%, nuts intake $< 10g/day$ in 41.81%, dairy products intake $< 300g/day$ in 65.95%, meats intake $< 100g/day$ in 36.54%, and seafood intake $< 100g/day$ in 88.75%. The synthesized data also showed inadequate energy intake in the respondents and unbalanced macronutrients distribution with 46.67% of daily calories from carbohydrates and 35.37% from fats. Despite sufficient consumption of protein, iron and niacin, ingestion of many other vitamins and minerals was below the recommended dietary allowance (RDA), especially for vitamin A, vitamin C, zinc, and selenium. The healthcare workers' unhealthy eating behaviors were interpreted to be contributing factors to the unbalanced dietary ingestion. In particular, healthcare workers who ate away from home (eating at home for $< 7times/week$), ate irregularly or had short mealtime ($< 30minutes$) had a higher risk of dietary inadequacy than those who ate regularly at home. Still, those who brought home-made meals to work were less likely to have inadequate intake of vitamin A, vitamin B2, calcium, and potassium than those who went to cafeterias or restaurants ($P < 0.05$).

The finding in this cross-sectional survey about Chinese healthcare workers' health status and dietary habits was worrisome. Although many medical staffs in the survey had substantial self-awareness about the health issues and a willingness to maintain a healthy diet, they need to take more actions. The high-intensity workplace to some extent was not staff-friendly enough for the workers to take care of their own health, and establishing a supportive nutritional service system is of necessity. In 2020, the Chinese National Health Commission commenced the "Healthy Canteens" initiative to ensure provision of adequate nutrients to healthcare workers optimize, occupational health of them, and thereby improve the health and well-being of people all around the nation.

As for the hospital managers, awareness should be raised about the healthcare staffs' life quality and mental status, necessary policies be issued and services be provided to improve the staff's working conditions, health status and guarantee their access to a healthy and nutritious diet. On the other hand, the healthcare workers should improve their own eating habits and become more health conscious. In general, working in the fields of health science, doctors should pay attention to healthy eating themselves, which plays an important role in realizing the vision of "Healthy China 2030".

References

［1］Report on Chinese Residents' Chronic Diseases and Nutrition (2020). Chinese State Council. December 23, 2020. Available online: http://www.gov.cn/xinwen/2020-12/24/content_5572983.htm

［2］Healthy China (2019－2030). Healthy China Action Promotion Committee. July 9, 2019. Available online: http://www.gov.cn/xinwen/2019-07/15/content_5409694. htm

［3］Chinese Doctor Diet Report. Meituan. August 18, 2020. Available online: https://ishare.ifeng.com/c/s/v002tGQzZjf9e9Shg6-_fxIMOwzQeOS8yIOYqg27--4MXZ78I

［4］Zhu XR. Investigation on Dietary Habits and Nutrition Intake of Emergency ICU Medical Staffs. World Latest Med 2018; 18: 11-2.

［5］The Writing Committee of the Report on Cardiovascular Health and Diseases in China. Interpretation of Report on Cardiovascular Health and Diseases in China 2019. Chin J Cardiovasc Med 2020; 35: 833-54.

[6] Scientific Research Report on Dietary Guidelines for Chinese (2021). Chinese Nutrition Society 2020. Available online: https://www.cnsoc.org/learn-news/422120203.html

[7] U.S. Department of Agriculture and U.S. Department of Health and Human Services. Dietary Guidelines for Americans, 2020－2025. 9th Edition. December 2020. Available online: https://www.dietaryguidelines.gov/sites/default/files/2020-12/Dietary_Guidelines_for_ Americans_2020-2025.pdf

[8] Chinese Nutrition Society. Chinese Dietary Guidelines (2016). Beijing: People's Medical Publishing House, 2016: 115-6.

主编导读（二）

女性，是否适合从事外科医生职业？

经历了几十年的临床外科生涯以后，深深体会到医生这项工作是一个拼体力、拼脑力、还拼持久力的活儿，实在是不好干。身负患者的生命重任，责任自然是天一样大。

很年轻的时候，我曾经问过我的澳大利亚外科老师 Donald Beard 为什么在西方国家外科医生收入那么高，他答道：世界上高收入的职业无外乎以下三种类型，要么是从事该工作需要经受很长时间、很严格的培训，一般人短期学习干不了的；要么是这个工作风险性很高，动不动危及生命的（如飞行员、间谍）；还有就是这个工作劳动强度非常大、特别累的，非高薪没人肯干的。外科医生这个职业把上面的三点都占全了，世界上能真正做好这个工作的人实际上并不多。

这些年的工作中，身边有不少女性外科医生，她们在工作上跟男性外科医生不让须眉、各顶半边天，实在是感到她们特别不容易。我私下里的疑问是：女性，基于其独特的生理和心理特点，又有家庭和孩子的额外负担，到底是否应该或者适合从事这个职业？一方面，把如花般的女性安排在这个残酷的岗位上是不是心太狠、不够人道？另一方面，这个需要超强应急能力、过人体力和随叫随到的工作，是不是非常不适合女性来担当呢？

实际上这个想法在我的脑海里已经很久，但是说出来不免有性别歧视之嫌，而且评判女性是不是适合做外科医生，最有发言权的不是我们男性，而是女性外科医生本身。

于是，我特地向浙江大学附属第一医院的著名外科女教授白雪莉约了稿子，来谈一谈这个话题。当时我有言在先，什么意见、观点都可以展示，什么牢骚或后悔都可以吐槽。实际上我当时暗中期待着一篇有不少怨言的评论文章，并且还有可能规劝姐妹们最好离这个工作远点……但是接到白教授的文章，匆匆看完，着实让我震撼了一下，同时马上又觉得我体会和领悟到了现代女性内心的坚强，不是柔弱、纤细的外表所能够遮掩住的。满满的正能量使我对于现在中国女性外科医生刮目相看。

我特别希望欧美的外科同行们能够听到我们中国女外科医生心声，供国内的同行们进行交流。

我知道各个地区、各个层面的女外科医生们一定会有不同的声音，或者截然不同的感受，因为各自的处境和境遇相差很远，我们非常欢迎大家发声。

女子不弱，为医益强——一个中国女外科医生眼中的性别属性

白雪莉

浙江大学附属第一医院　肝胆胰外科

"女子本弱，为母则刚"，乍看之下，说得很有道理。该句的作者是19世纪的男性，我没办法穿越回一百多年前看看那时候女性的生存状态，但是大概的印象是女性应该都没有工作，不需要上班，在家里相夫教子是她们的本分，而成为母亲就更像一种天职，更何谈女性参与医疗行业了。今天，我想说的是"女子不弱，为医益强"。

在日复一日的繁忙里，尤其是当手持手术刀站在无影灯下时，我会忘记自己女性的身份。但我又时时刻刻可以感受到，性别这一生理属性，在各个层面上为我外科医生这一职业身份带来的影响。

我相信，肯定不止我一个女外科医生时不时地会思考以下类似问题：在外科医生这个职业中，为何要谈论性别属性？女外科医生有哪些优势和劣势？如何成长为一名优秀的女外科医生？

今天，我试着通过20多年外科生涯的所见、所闻、所感，给出自己的答案。

在外科医生这个职业中，为何要谈论性别属性？

200多年前，对女外科医生的先驱者来说，谈论性别属性，可能是一个"生存，还是毁灭"的问题。出生在1789年的Margaret Ann Bulkley被认为是英国第一位女外科医生，但在超过40年的职业生涯中，她一直伪装成没有胡子的James Miranda Steuart Barry医生，直到1865年她的尸检报告公布时，人们才发现，她其实是个女人。

2019年，全球影响力最大的肿瘤学会——美国临床肿瘤学会的大会主席Monica M. Bertagnolli，是来自美国哈佛医学院附属布莱根和妇女医院肿瘤外科的女外科医生，也是哈佛大学医学院终身教授。同样是在2019年，中国医师协会外科医师分会发布《中国女性外科医师执业现状调查报告》。调研对象分布于30个省、自治区、直辖市及海外地区，结果显示，女性占外科医生总数的6.04%。她们的专业则主要集中在：甲状腺/乳腺外科（35.61%）、胃肠外科（19.55%）、肝胆胰外科（13.67%）。

200多年来，女外科医生，筚路蓝缕，砥砺前行，确实有令人欣喜的变化，但我们也应该看到，局限性也依然存在。女外科医生身上的性别枷锁是否已被打破？答案不言自明。事实证明，即使有这样那样的偏见，那也只是行进过程中的小障碍而已。"当你拿起手术刀时，你没有性别，你就是医生。"

女外科医生有哪些优势和劣势

我在上课的时候，也有女生问我，作为一名女外科医生，会面临什么样的压力？其实这个问题，可以细化为女性选择外科医生这个职业，有哪些优势和劣势？具体到个人，如何判断自己适不适合呢？

《中国女性外科医师执业现状调查报告》（2019年）显示，多数女外科医生认为，自己在从事外科方面，较男性存在一些劣势，如体力、生理、家庭等方面。但从优势上讲，她们多数认为：自己心思更加细腻、思虑周全、操作更轻柔灵活、损伤更小且对待患者更有耐心。

医学界这些年也做过一些有意思的研究，如《英国医学杂志》发表的一项研究中，对2007—2015年在加拿大安大略省接受手术的10.4万余名患者进行回顾性队列研究，探讨外科医生性别对普通外科手术患者术后效果的影响。其中一个颇具争议的结论是，女外科医生的患者比男外科医生的患者在手术30天后死亡的可能性要低4%；在再入院和并发症方面，则没有显著差异。

女医生比男医生更能以患者为中心进行交流，女医生通常花更长的时间问诊，征求患者的意见，并提供更多的心理问题、生活方式、日常生活、社会关系、压力与应对策略有关的咨询。当患者表示需要时，她们更能表达同情、关心和安慰，研究者认为这与良好的治疗效果存在不可分割的联系。

如何成长为一名优秀的女外科医生？

强烈的发心、对治病救人强烈的渴望、在每一个"十字路口"可以说是执拗的坚持、持续不断的学习、回溯个人经历，这几点但凡缺一点，我可能都成不了一名女外科医生，更不要说优秀。所以最终，我们要讨论的问题应该回归到：如何成为一名优秀的女外科医生？

首先，兴趣是最好的导师

走上从医这条道路，并非反复考量权衡利弊后的选择，更是一种自然而然的结果。在高考填写志愿的时候，我没有和任何人商量，全部填报了医学专业，带着一种不成功便成仁的轴劲。当年填志愿时，虽然有强烈的初心，但对外科乃至医学这门学科，我并没有直观的概念。

如今，外科这门学科或者说这个职业，已经向我展现出无与伦比的魅力，在错综复杂的症状中寻找本质、在迷宫一般的脉管中发现手术的空间、在不可能中捕获可能，都会让我兴奋异常，并且沉醉其中。这么多年过去了，这种对专业的强烈兴趣依然如初。这应该是外科医生成长之路上首要的，也是最大的驱动力。

其次，专注是冲破一切阻碍的钻头

和男医生相比，女外科医生要面对的阻碍更多。2015年，《美国医学会杂志》发表的一项研究表明，女医生比男医生在学术界更难达到正教授级别（11.9% vs 28.6%）。

2020年3月，南方周末报社发布《中国医护从业人员职业现状调研》，结果显示，女性在同岗位竞争中的压力明显大于男性。这些职业道路上的阻碍，促使我们格外需要具备坚持和专注。为了保持这种专注，我们很多时候不得不亏欠家庭，尤其是对于孩子的成长，没有什么参与感，从内心来说是愧疚的。

此外，领导力是从一个成功迈向另一个成功的关键

要做一个优秀的女外科医生，从一开始，从小决策开始，就应该日复一日磨炼自己的领导力。要想增强领导力，还要内外兼修，要主动发挥内在的力量、培育能促进职业发展的环境，并注重增强适应力以及适时调整工作状态。我希望更多优秀的青年加入到我们的队伍中来，不论性别，只看优秀与否。

外科医生是极其辛苦和需要承受极大压力的职业，但它也会带给你同样程度，甚至更加强烈的愉悦。而得到这种回报的前提是，你的发心是什么？

只有真正的热爱，才能够保持专注，才能具备直面困难的勇气。这颗心是一粒种子，决定了以后结出什么样的果实。

参考文献

［1］Park A. Researchers find women make better surgeons than men. TIMES, 2017-10-10.

［2］Chen PW. Do women make better doctors? The New York Times, 2010-05-06.

［3］Jena AB, Khullar D, Ho O, et al. Sex differences in academic rank in US medical schools in 2014. JAMA 2015; 314: 1149-58.

［4］Columbus AB, Lu PW, Hill SS, et al. Factors associated with the professional success of female surgical department chairs: a qualitative study. JAMA Surg 2020; 155: 1028-33.

A female surgeon's thoughts on gender attributes in surgery

Bai Xueli

Department of Hepatobiliary and Pancreatic Surgery, The First Affiliated Hospital, Zhejiang University School of Medicine, Hangzhou, China

There is a Chinese old saying that started in the 19th century: "A woman is vulnerable, but being a mother makes one strong". This seems to make sense, considering the status of women in society around a hundred years ago. None of us lived in that period, but we can imagine that women who lived back then might not have been obligated to work or assume a profession. Rather, it seemed more natural for them to do housework and teach their children at home. Being a mother is more like a sworn duty, perhaps similar to that of a doctor in the medical field. When I reflect on modern society, what I want to say is "women are not vulnerable, participating in medicine makes one stronger".

Each busy day, especially when standing on the operating table with a scalpel in my hand, I forget my identity as a woman. Apart from these moments, however, the impact of the identity and physiological attributes of being female permeate my profession as a surgeon.

I am certain that I am not the only female surgeon to wonder about the following questions from time to time: why should we talk about gender attributes in surgeons? What are the advantages and disadvantages of being a female surgeon? How do you become an excellent female surgeon?

Here, I am trying to answer these questions based on what I have seen, heard, and felt during the two decades of my surgical career.

Q1: Why should we talk about gender attributes in surgeons?

For the pioneer female surgeons of 200 years ago, this issue of being a woman and a surgeon was one of "to be, or not to be". Born in 1789, Margaret Ann Bulkley was considered to be the first female surgeon in the United Kingdom, but during the four decades of her surgical career, she disguised herself as the "beardless" James Miranda Steuart Barry. It was not until her autopsy report in 1865 that it was revealed she was actually a woman.

Over the past 200 years, women have made progress in the field of medicine. In 2019, the chief of the American Society of Clinical Oncology, the most influential oncology society in the world, was Dr. Monica M. Bertagnolli. Dr. Bertagnolli is a woman and a tenured professor of surgery at Harvard Medical School and chief of the Division of Surgical Oncology at Brigham and Women's Hospital. However, the same year, the Chinese College of Surgeons published the "Investigation Report on the Practice Status of Chinese Female Surgeons" [2019]. This investigation included surgeons from 30 different provinces, municipalities, autonomous regions, and countries. The results showed that women accounted for only 6.04% of the total number of surgeons. The majority of them were in thyroid and breast surgery (35.61%), gastrointestinal surgery (19.55%), and hepatobiliary and pancreatic surgery (13.67%).

Over the past two centuries, female surgeons have striven to move forward. There have been indeed been many positive changes made in the surgical field, but the lingering limitations should be recognized. Gender discrimination still plays a role in the careers of female surgeons, but this obstacle will soon be overcome: "A person who holds the scalpel in hand

守在生命的边缘
医者沉思录

is a surgeon, regardless of their gender".

Q2: What are the advantages and disadvantages of being a female surgeon?

Many female medical students ask me what kind of difficulties I face as a female surgeon. However, I think this question can be reframed in terms of what the advantages and disadvantages are of being a female surgeon, and a consideration on the individual level about how one decides whether he or she is suitable for this career.

The "Investigation Report on the Practice Status of Chinese Female Surgeons" [2019] showed that most female surgeons felt that they were at a disadvantage in terms of physical strength, family obligations, etc. In terms of advantages, most of them believed that they were more patient, considerate, and dexterous, and were able to injure patients less during operations than male surgeons.

Other interesting research has been conducted in this field over the years. A paper published in the British Medical Journal retrospectively analyzed a cohort of more than 104,000 patients who underwent surgery in Ontario, Canada from 2007 to 2015. The goal was to investigate whether the gender of surgeons played a role in general surgical outcomes. One controversial result was that the perioperative mortality rate of patients of female surgeons was 4% lower than that of patients with male surgeons. However, in terms of hospital readmissions and surgical complication rates, these two groups showed no significant differences [1].

In addition, female doctors tend to have more patient-centered communication. They usually spend more time with patients, asking patient opinions, and are more encouraging and reassuring when patients experience difficulties in mental health, lifestyle modification, social relations, or coping with stress [2]. I believe these qualities are essential to good patient care.

Q3: How to become an excellent female surgeon?

Looking back on my personal experience, if it were not for my strong desire to help patients and my motivation to learn continuously, I never would have become a female surgeon, let alone an excellent female surgeon.

Thus, the question comes back to "how does one become an excellent female surgeon?".

First, my interest in medicine was the biggest driving force to succeeding in my career. When I filled out my college applications, I did not discuss my choices with anyone because all applications were for programs in medicine. It was a natural choice and not the result of weighing the pros and cons of different options: I did not want to go into any major if it was not medicine. I actually did not know much about surgery or the medical field at that time, despite having a pure passion for medicine. Today, however, I can identify the diseases from insidious symptoms, find operative spaces between numerous tiny vessels and nerves, and make the impossible become possible. The magic of the surgical profession has engrossed me for decades and my passion for this career has never wavered. This is why I believe that being passionate about medicine is the most important driving force for becoming a surgeon.

Secondly, one must be fully dedicated to medicine to overcome any obstacles. Compared with our male colleagues, female surgeons tend to face more challenges in their careers. In 2015, a study published in the *Journal of the American Medical Association* showed that female doctors were less likely to become tenured professors than were male doctors (11.9% vs. 28.6%) [3]. Another study *"Survey on the Occupational Status of Chinese Healthcare Workers"* published by the Southern Weekly in March 2020 stated that women were facing greater pressure

| 守在生命的边缘
医者沉思录

than were men who worked in the same position. A great portion of this pressure comes from having to balance the obligations of career and family, and thus female surgeons need to be extremely persistent and resilient on their career path in order to manage these problems and find an equilibrium.

Last but not least, leadership is the key to become an outstanding surgeon. To be an exceptional female surgeon, one should participate in the decision-making process, even for minor issues. One should also take initiative, foster a healthy working environment, and be adaptive to different situations [4].

I truly hope that more outstanding young people can join our team, regardless of gender. Being a surgeon is an extremely hard and stressful profession, but it can also bring an equal or greater amount of joy. The main prerequisite for this career is that one know what one is truly passionate about. Only people with a true love for medicine can be fully dedicated to this career and have the courage to face all of its difficulties. This love is a seed, which determines what kind of fruit will blossom in the future.

References

[1] Park A. Researchers find women make better surgeons than men. TIMES, 2017-10-10.

[2] Chen PW. Do women make better doctors? The New York Times, 2010-05-06.

[3] Jena AB, Khullar D, Ho O, et al. Sex differences in academic rank in US medical schools in 2014. JAMA 2015; 314: 1149-58.

[4] Columbus AB, Lu PW, Hill SS, et al. Factors associated with the professional success of female surgical department chairs: a qualitative study. JAMA Surg 2020; 155: 1028-33.

主编导读（三）

医者不能自医？医生的心理健康，谁来关注……

医生的存在就是为了解除患者的疾患，包括疾病带来的身体痛苦，以及造成的心理上的压力和挫折。医生被教育和鼓励去减轻患者的焦虑和心理压力，使得他们能更好地了解疾病、更坦然地面对疾病。在接受医学治疗后，患者不仅得到身体上的康复，在心理上也能有良好的调理。

无论是公众还是医务人员，都认同解除或减轻患者的身心痛苦是医生的职责，并以此来作出要求或自我要求。但是，医生是一项身心压力均很大的职业，他们从事的是高风险、高强度的工作，日常工作中稍有不慎，可能就有生命的代价。而医务人员并非绝缘于社会之外，从个人层面看，普通人的痛苦和烦恼，如工资待遇、考核晋升、子女教育、老人赡养、家庭矛盾等，他们也都要一一面对。医务人员也吃五谷杂粮，身体也会出这样或那样的问题，他们中不少人也有自己的病痛。从社会层面看，社会的快速进步和发展让人眼花缭乱，并带来很多具冲击感的变迁和动荡，这些都会给人们的心理造成不同程度的震荡，这些因素给医务人员的心理冲击也是很大的，所以，医务人员承受着职业和社会的双重压力。

医生不是超人，不是从天而降拯救患者的神仙，他们最基本的属性是一个社会人。实际上，医务人员中存在着远超我们想象的抑郁和倦怠现象。近年来，国际上对于医务人员的抑郁和职业倦怠问题有了比较热烈的讨论，但国内还鲜有关注。这个问题必须得到重视，我们觉得至少有两个层面的含义：第一，医务人员在给患者解除病痛、减轻精神压力之外，也需要注意调节和治疗自身的压力和抑郁问题，使得自身能在足够健康的心理状态下工作；第二，只有当给患者治病的医务人员心理状态也处于良好水平时，才有可能更好地为患者服务。当自己心情极其低落、非常烦躁、出现抑郁的情况下，是很难耐心、细致地为患者看病的。

是时候关注医务人员尤其是中国医务人员的身心健康了！这是一个重要但长期被忽略的问题，我们首先需要了解它，对此进行有益的讨论，并且做出认真的应对计划和方案。也呼吁卫生主管部门能够更加重视医务人员心理健康问题，并采取相应的措施。

　　自从1991年尼泊尔提交了第一个世界精神卫生日报告以来，每年的10月10日被规定为世界精神卫生日。至今年（注：指2021年）正好是30周年纪念，借此之机，*HBSN*杂志专门邀请了新加坡心理卫生学院的Kelvin Lin Chieh Ng教授和北京和睦家医院心理学家刘辰博士共同撰写了一篇有关医务人员心理健康的文章。

你永远不会独行：
医疗专业人员的职业倦怠与抑郁

吴麟杰[1] 刘 辰[2]

[1]新加坡精神卫生研究所
[2]北京和睦家医院

流行病有三波浪潮：感染和死亡、社会经济的重创，以及疫情对公众心理的冲击。COVID-19的全球性大流行已导致2亿余人感染，各种经济和社会的紧张形势也见诸报道。同时，研究发现，在流行病暴发及之后的一段时期，群众和医疗专业人员都面临更多的心理健康问题。

有身心健康才是真正的健康

健康的定义随着时间的推移而改变，我们过去只关注生物模型，视健康为身体的正常功能状态。WHO在后期认识到健康应与幸福联系起来，并将健康定义为身体、心理和社会方面的良好状态，而不仅仅是没有疾病。

躯体疾病与精神疾病：同等与不平等

2010年，包括物质滥用在内的精神问题占全球疾病负担的10.4%。2011年，世界经济论坛发表言论提到精神疾病的隐藏成本（1.7万亿美元）远高于其造成的直接经济损失，尽管精神障碍比慢性病（如糖尿病）占用更高的经济成本，然而精神障碍的诊断和治疗程度却与其他专科差距甚大。社会认为心理健康对生活和福祉非常重要，但在治疗方面，我们仍侧重于解决躯体而非精神问题。

抑郁症：医疗工作者不能免疫

抑郁症是世界范围内的常见疾病，有超过2.64亿人受其影响，相当于世界人口的3.4%。多项研究表明，与一般人群相比，医学生和住院医师的抑郁症患病率为15%～30%，即使在职业生涯的成熟期，他们也不能免于患病。

实际上，医生不仅不能对抑郁症免疫，也正是医生的某些特点，使他们更容易罹患抑郁症。作为医生，他们面临工作、行政、教学、科研的多重压力。睡眠剥夺、牺牲饭点和如厕时间，即使在家里，也时常忧心工作的事情。年轻医生要忍受跑腿和杂活、随叫随到、各种考核、经常值班，并寄希望于成为专家后情况会好转。有些专家反过来羡慕年轻医生的自由，比如具有特定手术技术的人，抱怨自己成了专业知识和效率的奴隶。

专业精神和完美主义

行医不仅要遵守国家的法律，而且还要遵循更高的道德标准和专业精神。网络舆论会因为医生的道德瑕疵或犯罪行为迅速发酵，如果始作俑者是工程师或建筑师，似乎不会受到这种"隆重"的待遇。

除了法律、道德规范和专业精神，他们更受到自己内心的约束。很多医生具备一些品质，比如高标准和充满动力，他们不断自我提升、挑战极限……这些品质驱使他们成为更优秀的医学专家。不幸的是，事实证明，完美主义、自我苛求等这些在医生群体中常有的优秀品质，会增加个人罹患抑郁症的风险。他们从医是为了帮助他人和挽救生命，但遗憾的是，他们面对死亡常常无能为力。面对这样的"失败"时，那些刚刚提及的他们所具备的品质可能会让他们出现严重的自我怀疑甚至过度自责，他们甚至无法考虑这种失败是由于其他原因或不可控的外力造成，但这种倾向对个人的自尊和价值感产生严重的负面影响。

医者自医之？医者不自医

自己治疗自己总是存在风险的。首要的原因是，人很难清楚认识困扰自身的问题。就像我们在治疗家人亲友时无法完全客观，要么因为个人原因不能周全考虑和鉴别诊断，要么无法保持职业和亲情间的界限。很多时候，我们忽视各种迹象和症状，用理由和数字敷衍自己，希望问题赶紧自行消失，结果却拖到为时已晚的地步。

即便我们下定决心不再拖延，我们也很少为自己的病情寻求规范的评估和治疗，尤其是涉及个人心理健康的问题。有好几次我的同行医生们在走道和电梯里替他们的"朋友或患者"向我咨询关于抑郁量表和药物治疗的问题，他们实际上可能是在为自己寻找这些问题的答案。很多时候，他们避免向同事暴露自己的弱点，尝试为自己治疗，希望情况获得改善，也许他们可以用某种办法解决咳嗽、感冒这样的小问题，但抑郁症和其他心理障碍的治疗并不是那么简单直接的，疾病会削弱一个人的判断力、行动力和自制力，而自我治疗有时会造成更大的伤害。

社会污名化，医疗专业人员的偏见，还有自我歧视

WHO将污名定义为一种羞耻或负面的印象，导致个人被拒绝、歧视和被社会诸多领域排斥。抑郁症作为一种精神障碍，与之相关的污名依然非常严重，我们知道精神疾病患者的社会性歧视是治疗过程中的主要障碍。医生可能通过一些方面表现出对精神疾病的拒斥：他们可能对患者的心理健康史不感兴趣，对治疗持悲观态度，对诊断和相关信息交流不足，或在精神疾病的治疗安排和康复计划上存在结构性的偏见。

这种与精神问题相关的羞耻感也影响了医疗专业人员在心理健康问题上寻求帮助的意愿，他们害怕被认为能力不足、效率低下、不可靠甚至不安全，因此拖延和隐藏问题就不足为奇了。另外就是来自外部原因的担忧，比如医院或者卫生管理机构可能会（无论是真实的还是假设）对存在心理健康问题的医生产生偏见，进而影响

他们的职业发展和机会，尽管他们的心理健康问题没有对执业能力造成损害。

也许更具破坏性的是医疗工作者对自身心理问题的偏见。自我污名化涉及情感上或认知上吸收关于自我的负面信念，感到羞耻，自我认同感很低，加之对精神疾病的刻板印象，从而疏远他人、对自己亦感到无能为力。指出可能有抑郁症等心理健康问题，无论是对同行，还是对我们自己来说，都会被担心造成尴尬、不适和伤害。这种自我污名化剥夺了我们寻求专业帮助的机会，也剥夺了治愈的可能。

结论：不为知识而骄傲，但因智慧而谦卑

"不为知识而骄傲，但因智慧而谦卑"是我第一次踏入医学院就学到的校训。简单来说，这意味着作为医学生，随着知识的增长和学术的进步，我们应该始终保持谦逊的态度。然而，当我写下这些结束语时，在更广泛的语境下，我再次想起了母校的座右铭。我们有多少次建议、鼓励甚至告诫我们的患者要照顾好自己，吃好睡好、休息好，告诉他们生病时要善待自己；而当谈到自己时，我们却无视这些？我们拥有专业的知识和临床技能，正是这种骄傲反而使我们不愿遵循正确的建议。或许我们都需要学会谦虚，首先看到我们作为人类个体，在生理和心理上，拥有人性的弱点和患病的脆弱；然后我们再专注于知识技能，最终获得帮助自己和别人的大智慧。

参考文献

［1］Whiteford HA, Degenhardt L, Rehm J, et al. Global burden of disease attributable to mental and substance use disorders: findings from the Global Burden of
Disease Study 2010. Lancet 2013; 382: 1575-86.

［2］Bloom DE, Cafiero ET, Jané-Llopis E, et al. The global economic burden of non-
communicable diseases. Geneva: World Economic Forum, 2011.

［3］GBD 2017 Disease and Injury Incidence and Prevalence Collaborators. Global, regional, and national incidence, prevalence, and years lived with disability for 354 diseases and injuries for 195 countries and territories, 1990－2017: a systematic analysis for the Global Burden of Disease Study 2017. Lancet. 2018; 392: 1789-858. Erratum in: Lancet 2019; 393: e44.

［4］Tyssen R, Vaglum P, Grønvold NT, et al. Suicidal ideation among medical students and young physicians: a nationwide and prospective study of prevalence and predictors. J Affect Disord 2001; 64: 69-79.

［5］Vaillant GE, Sobowale NC, McArthur C. Some psychological vulnerabilities of physicians. N Engl J Med 1972; 287: 372-5.

［6］Heim E, Kohrt BA, Koschorke M, et al. Reducing mental health-related stigma in primary healthcare settings in low-and middle-income countries: a systematic review. Epidemiol Psychiatr Sci 2018; 29: e3.

［7］Knaak S, Mantler E, Szeto A. Mental illness-related stigma in healthcare: Barriers to access and care and evidence-based solutions. Healthc Manage Forum 2017; 30: 111-6.

［8］Henderson C, Noblett J, Parke H, et al. Mental health-related stigma in health care and mental health-care settings. Lancet Psychiatry 2014; 1: 467-82.

You shall never walk alone: burnout and depression amongst healthcare professionals

Kelvin Lin Chieh Ng[1], Liu Chen[2]

[1]Institute of Mental Health, Singapore, Singapore
[2]United Family Hospital, Beijing, China

Introduction

There are two stages of tsunami, first is the earthquake in deep sea, followed by hurricane. There are three waves of pandemic, the death toll, economic and social disruption, and a psychological storm that is looming in the distance nowadays. In this time of worldwide COVID-19 pandemic, to date, we have seen over 200 million cases worldwide, and the death toll is in excess of 4 million, and there are various news reports coming in about devastating economic and social situation. Moreover, numerous studies report that the public, as well as the healthcare professionals are at heightened risk mental health problems in the short and longer term from pandemic.

There is no health without mental health

Definitions of health have changed throughout time, we used to just focus on the biological model, and health then was seen as a state of normal function of the body that could be disrupted from time to time by disease. The World Health Organization in later years, has recognized the importance of linking health to well-being instead, and has defined health as "a state of complete physical, mental and social well-being and not merely the absence of disease and infirmity".

Equality, or rather, inequality between physical and mental illness

In 2010, it was noted that mental and substance use disorders constituted 10.4% of the global burden of disease, and were the leading cause of years lived with disability amongst all disease groups [1]. In 2011, the World Economic Forum acknowledged that there are "hidden costs" of diseases (US$1.7 trillion), which are much higher than the direct costs [2], that has made mental disorders accounted for more economic costs than chronic physical diseases such as cancer or diabetes, yet, the treatment gap for mental disorders is higher than for any other health sector. Thus, the system sees the increasing importance of mental and social well-being to be considered as an integral part of health, but strives to attain and achieve on top of just physical health.

We are not immune

Depression is a common illness worldwide, with more than 264 million people affected and this is estimated to be equivalent to 3.4% of the world's population [3]. There are several robust studies which have suggested that the rates of depression are higher in medical students and residents (15%－30%) as compared to the general population, and this pattern seems to persist even despite the advancement of their professional career [4].

We have to understand that physicians are not only not immune to depression, but we possess certain psychological vulnerabilities that make us more susceptible to depression. As doctors, we are often subjected to punishing work schedules, administrative procedures, teaching and training and research. We often have insufficient sleep, sometimes sacrificing our meals and toilet breaks, even at home, we are hardly getting rest without worrying about work. Junior doctors have to endure physical hardship of doing scud work and being on-call and passing the exams, with the hope that life will be better when they become specialists. Ironically, the experts in the field of practice find themselves envying the juniors for their freedom: specialist who is the only one able to perform a particular surgical procedure, and thus one becomes a slave to one's expertise and efficiency.

Professionalism and perfectionism

We know that the medical profession is not only subjected to the laws of the land wherewith we practice medicine, but we are also held accountable to an even higher standard of professionalism and clinical ethics. The tabloids and newspapers are quick to emblazon front page headlines of this doctor being found out of having an affair or guilty of some other sordid or sensational crime, but we certainly do not see such similar treatment if the perpetrator is an engineer or architect.

Apart from being held accountable to the legal system, the clinical code of ethics and professionalism, many of us are perhaps most bound by ourselves. Many doctors possess certain qualities, like ambition and drive, setting high standards for themselves, that make us to be the best that we can be, to push ourselves to our absolute peak and to challenge our limits, and these qualities drive us to become excellent doctors. Unfortunately, it is proven that those personality traits like perfectionism and self-criticism are common among physicians, which increase the risk of depression [5]. We enter into Medicine to help people and save lives, but more often than not, sadly, we face failure and loss. When facing such "failure", it is the same qualities that we value may lead us to self-doubt and worse, self-criticism and self-blame, personal responsibility overshadows all else and we are not even able to consider whether there were other mitigating factors or extenuating circumstances that could have contributed to the failure, and this can be extremely damaging to one's self-esteem and pride.

Physician, heal thyself! Or should we?

There is always the danger that we as doctor face, when it comes to caring for ourselves. Many of us are first blind to what ails us. Just like we are not able to be objective when it comes to treating our family and loved ones, either fearing to consider more serious diagnoses because we do not wish for such a condition to be present, or else we are not able to distance ourselves to our loved ones when it is required to administer treatment, like operating on their bodies, so it is when it comes to ourselves. Very often, we ignore signs and symptoms, deceiving ourselves with facts and figures in the hope that it would go away, and end up seeking for help only when it is too late.

Even when we have decided that we can no longer ignore the problem, seldom do we seek formal consultation and treatment for our ailments, especially when it is mental health related. I recall there are times when I have been engaged in a "corridor consultation" with my other colleagues, asking on behalf of their "friend or patient", informally of course, about self-assessment tools, or other conversations on WeChat or WhatsApp about what is the treatment for Depression, and we know that they might actually be seeking these answers for themselves. Very often, we shy away from exposing ourselves or showing weakness to our fellow colleagues, and try to administer treatment for ourselves, in the hope of getting better without a formal medical review. I guess we can treat ourselves for minor ailments like coughs and colds, but the treatment of Depression and other mental illnesses are not so straightforward, as the illness impairs one's judgement, motivation and insight, and self-treatment can sometimes lead to more harm than good.

Stigma, stigma amongst healthcare professionals and self-stigma

WHO defined stigma as "a mark of shame, disgrace or disapproval that results in an individual being rejected, discriminated against and excluded from participating in a number of different areas of society". Depression, and indeed, mental illness as a whole, has a very great stigma associated with it, and we know that stigmatization of persons with mental illness is a major barrier in the treatment process. The doctors may exhibit stigma towards mental illness in one or more of the following ways: they may be disinterested in the patient's mental health history, become therapeutic pessimism, structural discrimination related to poor quality psychiatric treatment or rehabilitation measures and sharing insufficient information on diagnosis [6].

With such stigma associated with mental illness, it is thus not surprising that this stigma has also impacted healthcare professionals with regards to willingness to seek help for a mental health problem, for fear of being perceived as less competent, less productive and unsafe to work with even [7]. There is the added burden or worry that the healthcare institution may, either real or perceived, prejudice against those medical practitioners with mental health issues, and affect their career opportunities and further advancement, even though their mental health issue may not affect their ability to perform at work.

Perhaps more significant and damaging is that of self-stigma. Self-stigma involves emotionally or cognitively absorbing the negative beliefs about the self, largely based on shame, accepting mental illness stereotypes, alienating oneself from others, and feeling a sense of disempowerment [8]. We may feel embarrassed, or worse shame, to admit that we may be having a mental health issue like depression, either to another medical professional, or even ourselves. This self-stigma thus robs us of seeking professional help, and a chance of getting better.

Conclusions

Not pride of knowledge, but humility of wisdom

The school motto of *"Not Pride of Knowledge, but Humility of Wisdom"* was introduced to me when I first entered medical school. In simple terms, it meant that as medical students, as we progressed in our medical studies and gained knowledge, we should always remain humble. However, as I write these closing words, I am reminded again of my alma mater's motto, but applied in a different way. How often do we advise, encourage and sometimes admonish our patients to take care of themselves, to eat and sleep properly, to rest, to have self-care whenever they are sick, and ignore these words when it comes to ourselves? We have the knowledge, but it is our pride that keeps us from following our own advice. Perhaps we all need to be learn humility, to understand that we are but human, with all our human fragilities and weaknesses that make us prone to disease, physical or mental, and then only will we pay heed to our knowledge, and finally gain wisdom.

References

[1] Whiteford HA, Degenhardt L, Rehm J, et al. Global burden of disease attributable to mental and substance use disorders: findings from the Global Burden of Disease Study 2010. Lancet 2013; 382: 1575-86.

[2] Bloom DE, Cafiero ET, Jané-Llopis E, et al. The global economic burden of noncommunicable diseases. Geneva: World Economic Forum, 2011.

[3] GBD 2017 Disease and Injury Incidence and Prevalence Collaborators. Global, regional, and national incidence, prevalence, and years lived with disability for 354 diseases and injuries for 195 countries and territories, 1990－2017: a systematic analysis for the Global Burden of Disease Study 2017. Lancet. 2018; 392:

1789-858. Erratum in: Lancet 2019; 393: e44.

[4] Tyssen R, Vaglum P, Grønvold NT, et al. Suicidal ideation among medical students and young physicians: a nationwide and prospective study of prevalence and predictors. J Affect Disord 2001; 64: 69-79.

[5] Vaillant GE, Sobowale NC, McArthur C. Some psychological vulnerabilities of physicians. N Engl J Med 1972; 287: 372-5.

[6] Heim E, Kohrt BA, Koschorke M, et al. Reducing mental health-related stigma in primary healthcare settings in low-and middle-income countries: a systematic review. Epidemiol Psychiatr Sci 2018; 29: e3.

[7] Knaak S, Mantler E, Szeto A. Mental illness-related stigma in healthcare: Barriers to access and care and evidence-based solutions. Healthc Manage Forum 2017; 30: 111-6.

[8] Henderson C, Noblett J, Parke H, et al. Mental health-related stigma in health care and mental health-care settings. Lancet Psychiatry 2014; 1: 467-82.

让医患回暖

相热
关点

外科手术决策的宗旨只有一个：我们做的所有治疗，患者必须从中受益

从事外科工作这些年，我常暗中得意的是，好像没有一个学术界的专业人员能够像外科医生那样同时具备"学术"和"匠人"的双重特性。外科医生在学术上如果充分发挥专研，有可能成为一名科学家；同时在技术操作上如果精益求精，可能成为一个高超的"匠人"。而后者的"作品"可远远不局限在一个物件或者艺术作品，而是延长生命、减轻痛苦的效果。

外科专家可以是偏向学术型的，也同时可以是偏向手术操作型的，或者两者都具备。医生这个职业越想越是一个完美的结合体，是一个伟大的职业。可能世界上没有比这更好的职业了，这也解释为什么世界上有很多伟人出自外科医生，如切格瓦拉。

业界很多熟悉的、不熟悉的外科医生朋友沉醉在外科手术技巧中，可能不仅出于他们对于专业的责任和奉献，实际上还来自一个"匠人"对自己得意的"手艺活"的偏爱。他们如此努力，有很多原因并不完全源于经济和荣耀，而来自对于专业技巧的小得意，是一种别人做不了的但是我能做下来的心理满足和成就感。这也就是很多外科医生可以孜孜不倦地攻克外科新兴技术、高难技术的动力之一吧。

这样的心理，同时也可能造成一个问题：外科医生具有冲击技术极限和冒险的习惯，尤其体现在对于新的、高难技术的追求上面。外科医生有时可能会做一些技术上自己还没有充分把握的手术，当然这种精神使得外科界人才辈出、代有高手，但是可能客观上损害了患者的利益；另外，外科医生也可能因为"手术成瘾"，做一些本来不应该做的手术。

我们到底为了什么要做手术？我们必须回归到手术治疗的初衷上来，那就是所有的治疗包括外科治疗都是为了使患者经过治疗

能够从中获益而做的。这个获益包括了有效延长患者的生命，改善患者的生活质量，最大限度地减轻患者的痛苦。这点上我们应不忘初心。

当手术变成外科医生炫技、满足操作欲望的手法时，外科手术的方向就偏了。实际上，在挑战外科疑难手术幌子下我们有时确实做了超出自己技术范围和把握的手术；也有医生为了追求手术量而做一些患者不需要的手术。

偶然一次，我和我国著名的外科学家邢宝才教授共同看到一张幻灯片（见后面正文图），并就此进行过一些讨论，我们对此深有同感。我真诚邀请了邢宝才教授撰写一篇相关的论述。

外科手术决策的原则——患者获益了吗?

刘　明　邢宝才

北京大学肿瘤医院　肝胆胰外科Ⅰ科
北京大学肿瘤发生与转化研究教育部重点实验室

> "对于外科医生，上帝不可饶恕的两件事情是：
> 一是做自己没把握的手术；二是做患者不需要的手术。"
>
> ——马克斯·雷克
>
> *摩西·沙因编著《外科并发症的预防与处理》*
>
> For surgeons the Lord will not forgive these：
> 1.Do a surgery which they themselves are not confident of；
> 2.Operating on patients who do not need surgery.
>
> ——Max Thorek,
>
> In Moshe Schein edit：Prevention and Management of Surgical Complications

　　什么是外科手术？在繁忙的工作中，我们很难有时间去思考这个复杂的问题。一些超级医疗中心，收治患者、施行手术，已经成为流水线式的工作，当一台手术后患者恢复得很顺利、没有任何并发症的时候，我们暗自会对精湛的技艺沾沾自喜。但是，当患者出现严重的术后并发症甚至发生死亡的时候，我们不得不踩下刹车，进行一些思考：手术到底为患者带来了什么？

　　手术的目的是什么？哪些患者应该接受手术？其实，我们回顾外科手术的发展历史，就会发现这个问题有着清晰的答案。

最早的手术操作是为了帮助角斗士止血。随后，为了挽救战士的生命，医生发现必须进行截肢——这是早期最主要的手术类型。但我们可以想象，在只有烙铁、没有麻醉的情况下，在哀号中进行的截肢是一件多么恐怖的事情，以至于手术一度成为"野蛮"的代名词，这显然有悖于手术治疗的初衷。此后，医生们为了解决手术带来的痛苦而不懈努力，并逐渐奠定了外科的三大基石——麻醉、止血、消毒。此后，外科手术有了安全的保障，得以飞速发展，成为一种真正的治病方式。

随着手术安全性的明显提高，外科医生对解剖认识的深入、影像设备的更新与改进，以及手术器械的进步，外科手术的适应证逐渐扩大，进入大外科时代，过去许多仅存在于想象中的治疗方法今天都成为可能。比如我们曾经梦想能够让心脏停跳，打开心脏来为患者治疗心脏疾病，体外循环系统的发明使这种方法成为现实。肝炎、严重肝硬化造成的肝功能衰竭，外科医生可以通过肝移植来拯救患者的生命。而我们每年超过一万例的肾移植手术已经成为挽救尿毒症患者的成熟方法。

因此，手术是我们帮助患者的一种方式，每一次外科技术的进步及相关的麻醉、止血等方面的发展都是为了解决患者的需求。无论手术简单或复杂，都是为了使患者获益——要么延长患者的生存时间，要么提高患者的生活质量。实际上，这正是希波克拉底誓言的核心内容，即为患者谋利益，做自己力所能及的事情，绝不利用职业便利做道德缺失甚至违法的事情。诊疗活动中，我们牢记这些原则，就会使得很多决策变得简单容易。

此外，在手术安全性逐渐提高、外科技术快速发展的同时，外科医生应该清醒地认识到：手术是一把"双刃剑"，既可以帮助患者切除肿瘤，解除病痛，也会破坏患者躯体的完整性，造成机体的创伤，留下后遗症，甚至可能会危及生命。而且，医学的其他学科也在不断发展，内科药物的更新换代日新月异，治疗效果不断提高，例如肿瘤的免疫及靶向治疗，已经使患者的生存时间得到数倍延长。

所以，外科医生决定为患者实施手术前，必须认真思考以下两个问题。

（1）我们的外科手术能否给患者带来生存获益，或生活质量的改善。

（2）与其他学科的治疗方法相比，外科手术带来的生存获益是不是最大的；在同样获益的情况下，外科手术给患者的创伤是不是最小的。

要回答好这些问题，需要外科医生有持之以恒的学习习惯，丰富自己的知识。我们不仅要掌握外科领域的进步，还要充分了解其他学科的前沿进展。应该积极进行多学科诊疗，做到有所为，有所不为。

以结直肠癌肝转移（colorectal liver metastases，CRLM）为例，很多患者初始诊断的时候肝脏可能会有超过10个以上的转移病灶，有的患者甚至达到40～50个。这些患者应该积极转化还是姑息维持呢？大量的临床研究表明，CRLM是一类特殊的晚期疾病，具有良好的生物学特性，在系统治疗有效的前提下，以外科切除为主的局部治疗，如果能使患者达到NED状态（no evidence of disease state，无疾病状态），可以带来明显的生存获益。法国保罗布鲁斯医院Adam教授甚至提出这类患者的减瘤手术可能也是有意义的，所以这些患者的外科治疗应该更加积极，这就是所谓的有所为。

反之，同样作为晚期疾病，以胰腺癌肝转移为例，虽然今天的外科技术已经可以非常确切地切除所有肿瘤，通过胰十二指肠切除手术联合肝切除手术，使患者达到R0的状态，并且可以达到令人满意的手术安全性。但是，这类患者能够通过我们的手术延长生存时间吗？至少目前在没有有效的全身治疗药物的情况下，答案是否定的。因此这些患者不应该手术，或者说不应该首先选择手术。再比如，对于肝细胞性肝癌合并门静脉主干癌栓的患者，我们也可以安全达到R0切除，但这类患者接受手术的中位生存时间仅有6个月，而目前的免疫联合靶向治疗，生存时间也能够达到8个月，再联合放疗、介入治疗可以获得更长的生存时间，因此，对这部分患者直接进行手术也是不合适的。这就是所谓的有所不为。

再有，对于不可切除的胰头癌合并梗阻性黄疸的患者，解除黄疸是其首要问题。以前，我们通常给患者进行胆肠吻合手术。而如今，通过创伤很小的内镜技术植入支架就可以达到与外科手术同样的效果，因此，手术应该从这类患者的治疗方案中剔除。这也是所谓的有所不为。

因此，外科医生为了能给患者提出最合理的建议，一方面要不断填充自己的知识，做到博学多才，另一方面要积极参加并推动多学科诊疗。如果多学科诊疗团队中的每名医生都能够从患者利益出发，谨慎衡量自己手中的武器能够带给患者多少利益、会给患者造成多少弊害，那么无论结局如何，患者都已经得到了最佳治疗。

总之，作为外科医生应该谨记，手术的诞生与发展是为了解决患者的需求。以患者利益为中心是制定任何决策的基本原则，包括是否应该手术、什么时机手术以及如何进行手术的决策。单纯掌握外科技术已经不能成为一名合格的外科医生。我们要通过不断的学习、研究与合作，做到有所为及有所不为，力所能及，牢记初衷，砥砺前行。

参考文献

[1] Hippocrates. The oath. Available online: https://www.nlm. nih.gov/hmd/greek/greek_oath.html. June 15, 2019.

[2] Allard MA, Adam R, Giuliante F, et al. Long-term outcomes of patients with 10 or more colorectal liver metastases. Br J Cancer 2017; 117: 604-11.

[3] Adam R, Kitano Y, Abdelrafee A, et al. Debulking surgery for colorectal liver metastases: Foolish or chance? Surg Oncol 2020; 33: 266-9.

[4] Tempero MA, Malafa MP, Al-Hawary M, et al. Pancreatic Adenocarcinoma, Version 2. 2021, NCCN Clinical Practice Guidelines in Oncology. J Natl Compr Canc Netw 2021; 19: 439-57.

[5] Wang K, Guo WX, Chen MS, et al. Multimodality Treatment for Hepatocellular Carcinoma With Portal Vein Tumor Thrombus: A Large-Scale, Multicenter, Propensity Mathching Score Analysis. Medicine (Baltimore) 2016; 95: e3015.

[6] Moss AC, Morris E, Leyden J, et al. Malignant distal biliary obstruction: a systematic review and meta-analysis of endoscopic and surgical bypass results. Cancer Treat Rev 2007; 33: 213-21.

守在生命的边缘
医者沉思录

Surgical decision-making: can patients benefit?

Liu Ming, Xing Baocai

Key Laboratory of Carcinogenesis and Translational Research (Ministry of Education/Beijing), Hepatopancreatobiliary Surgery Department I, Peking University Cancer Hospital & Institute, Beijing, China

> For surgeons the Lord will not forgive these:
> 1.Do a surgery which they themselves are not confident of;
> 2.Operating on patients who do not need surgery.
>
> —Max Thorek,
>
> In Moshe Schein edit: Prevention and Management of Surgical Complications

What is surgery? It is difficult for us to have time to think about this broad question in our busy, day-to-day work. In some "super hospitals", patient admission and surgical operation have even become an "assembly-line" job. When a patient successfully recovers from an operation without any postoperative complications, we may be silently proud of our surgical skills. However, when the patient encounters serious postoperative complications or even death, we must pause and reflect: what does the operation bring to the patient? What is the purpose of an operation? What kind of patients should undergo surgery?

In fact, if we look back at the history of surgery, we can find clear answers to these questions.

The earliest known surgical operations were performed to stop the bleeding of injured gladiators. Later, doctors invented amputation in order to save soldiers' lives, which became the major type of operation in the early days. We can certainly imagine how terrifying an amputation could be when there was no anesthesia, with the operation being space filled with the patient's screams. Surgery was once a brutal exercise, which was obviously contrary to the original intention of surgical treatment. Since then, doctors have made unremitting efforts to relieve the surgery-related pain of patients. They gradually discovered the three principles of surgery—anesthesia, hemostasis, and disinfection—which ensured the safety of operations and enabled surgical techniques to develop rapidly. Surgery has thus become an effective medical treatment.

With the improvement of operation safety, surgeon's deeper understanding of anatomy, and the innovation of imaging equipment and surgical instruments, the indications of surgery have largely expanded, and we have now entered the era of surgery. Many previously unimaginable treatments have now become possible. For example, cardiac surgery was once considered impossible for patients with cardiac diseases because of the inability to stop the heart and operate. The creation of the cardiopulmonary bypass system made this dream a reality. Surgeons can also save patients with liver failure caused by hepatitis or severe cirrhosis through liver transplantation. Furthermore, kidney transplantation, with is completed in more 10,000 patients in China annually, has also matured as a treatment for patients with uremia.

Therefore, the ultimate goal of surgical operation is to help patients. All the developments of surgical techniques, including anesthesia, hemostasis, etc. are to serve the needs of patients. Regardless of whether an operation is simple or complex, the purpose of any operation is to benefit the patient, in either extending the patient's survival time or improving the patient's quality of life. This ethic is echoed in the core tenets of the Hippocratic oath: always come for the benefit of the sick and keep them from harm and injustice [1]. Through keeping the oath in mind, doctors can clarify and simplify many decision-making processes in their daily work.

Furthermore, as the safety of surgery and surgical technology rapidly improve and develop, surgeons should be increasingly cautious of surgery's "double-edged" nature: it can remove tumors and treat diseases but it can also affect the physical integrity of the patient's body, cause postoperative trauma and complications, and even lead to death. To minimize the negative aspects of surgery, surgeons need to know that other medical specialties are also rapidly developing. For example, in internal medicine, targeted therapy combined with immune therapy has prolonged the survival time of cancer patients by multiple times. Before deciding to perform surgery for the patient, surgeons must seriously consider the following two questions: (I) will the surgery bring survival benefits to the patient or improve the quality of life? (II) Compared with that of treatment from other medical specialties, is the survival benefit conferred by surgery the greatest? In cases of equal benefit, can surgery provide the least amount of injury to the patient?

To answer these questions, surgeons need to be persistent in learning and enriching their knowledge. Surgeons should not only be proficient within his/her own field of surgery but also keep abreast of the development of other fields. Multidisciplinary diagnosis and treatment (MDT) should be actively pursued because a good surgeon knows that "there are things that must be done and things that must not be done".

One example of what "must be done" is from colorectal liver metastasis (CRLM). Many patients may have more than 10 sites of CRLM when initially diagnosed, and some patients may even have 40-50 sites. Should these patients be treated actively or palliatively? A large number of clinical studies have shown that CRLM is a special type of advanced disease with good biological characteristics. On the premise that systemic treatment is effective, if patients can reach a no-evidence-of-disease state after surgical resection, patients can have significant survival benefits [2]. Professor Adam has even suggested that tumor reduction surgery for such patients may also be effective [3], so these patients should be actively treated with operation.

Conversely, an example of what "must not be done" is from pancreatic liver metastasis, which is also an advanced disease. Today's surgical techniques can remove all tumors accurately and safely, and patients can reach the R0 state via pancreaticoduodenectomy with liver resection. However, can these patients' survival time be prolonged through the surgery? In the absence of effective systemic therapy, the answer is no; thus, these patients should not have surgery [4] or should not consider surgery as their primary option. Another example of this is in patients with hepatocellular carcinoma with portal vein tumor thrombus, for whom the median survival time when undergoing surgery is only 6 months even when R0 resection is attained [5]; meanwhile, targeted therapy combined with immune therapy alone can attain 8 months of survival, and the median survival time can even be extended by combining radiation and interventional therapy. Therefore, in these patients, operation may not be appropriate.

Furthermore, in patients with unresectable pancreatic head cancer with obstructive jaundice, the primary goal is to resolve the jaundice. In the past, surgeons usually performed biliary-enteric anastomosis for these patients. Nowadays, minimally invasive endoscopic stenting can achieve the same effectiveness [6]. Surgery should also not be considered as the primary choice for these patients. This is another example of what "must not be done".

Therefore, in order to make the most appropriate suggestions to patients, surgeons must not only continue to learn and be knowledgeable but also actively participate in and promote MDT. If every doctor in the MDT team can think for the benefit of the patient and carefully weigh the advantages and disadvantages of the treatment plan, then, regardless of outcome, the patient has already received the best treatment possible.

In summary, surgeons should keep in mind that surgery was originally created and developed to meet the needs of patients. "Patient-centered treatment" is the basic principle for making any medical decision and can inform whether to operate, when to operate, and how to operate. A surgeon who simply masters the necessary surgical techniques cannot yet be recognized as a competent surgeon. We should continue to learn, conduct research, and cooperate with other specialists to understand "the things that must be done, and the things that must not be done". We must do the best we can, and move forward.

References

［1］ Hippocrates. The oath. Available online: https://www.nlm. nih.gov/hmd/greek/greek_oath.html. June 15, 2019.

［2］ Allard MA, Adam R, Giuliante F, et al. Long-term outcomes of patients with 10 or more colorectal liver metastases. Br J Cancer 2017; 117: 604-11.

［3］ Adam R, Kitano Y, Abdelrafee A, et al. Debulking surgery for colorectal liver metastases: Foolish or chance? Surg Oncol 2020; 33: 266-9.

［4］ Tempero MA, Malafa MP, Al-Hawary M, et al. Pancreatic Adenocarcinoma, Version 2. 2021, NCCN Clinical Practice Guidelines in Oncology. J Natl Compr Canc Netw 2021; 19: 439-57.

［5］ Wang K, Guo WX, Chen MS, et al. Multimodality Treatment for Hepatocellular Carcinoma With Portal Vein Tumor Thrombus: A Large-Scale, Multicenter, Propensity Mathching Score Analysis. Medicine (Baltimore) 2016; 95: e3015.

［6］ Moss AC, Morris E, Leyden J, et al. Malignant distal biliary obstruction: a systematic review and meta-analysis of endoscopic and surgical bypass results. Cancer Treat Rev 2007; 33: 213-21.

主编导读（五）

患者和家属是否应该参与医疗决策？

理论上说，针对患者各种疾病作出诊断、而后制定详细的治疗方案，这是医疗专业人员的专职和责任，因为专业的决定不应该受到医疗以外的任何因素的影响。就像我们坐飞机去外地，天气状况是否适合飞行、飞机的飞行速度和高度都是飞行人员根据专业规范和判断来定的，不会受旅客的要求或者意见所左右。这样才能够达到专业计划中最安全和良好效果。

但是医疗实践中，我们治疗的患者是活生生的有思想、有生活和社会背景的人群。患者和家属不但对于疾病需要有知情权，而且对于不同的治疗方案也有一定的选择权。人类是一个复杂的群体，有不同的生活和社会背景。对于主治医生为他们选择的治疗方案，患者可能会由于经济情况、所处的地域文化、自身对于疾病的认识、家庭关系，以及对于人生意义的理解不同而作出不同的选择。这些选择一般是在医生的专业建议基础上作出的，但又融合了各自的具体情况，医务人员还得尊重这些选择。

患者和家属对于医疗专业决定的介入深度，在中国和西方国家可能是不同的。这是因为文化、宗教和传统习惯不同，决定了很多处事方式不同。西方的患者一般会非常遵循医嘱；而中国患者和家属比较有意愿介入医疗决策中。这样就出现了一个问题，到底患者和家属应该多深地介入医疗决定？这个分寸没有规范、共识来界定，一般是由医患一起"摸着石头"决定的。如果医生的决定太过专断，不考虑到患者的家庭情况，那可能最后会出问题；同样如果治疗方案样样迁就患者，那么最佳的治疗措施不能得以执行，直接影响到患者的治疗效果。

现在，随着资讯的发达和检索的简易化，出现了一个新的现象。就是患者事先会就具体病种检索很多资料，做功课，然后一件件和专业医生核对。这种情况的好处是患者在就诊前对于具体病情有个初步的认识；坏处是有些网上的知识并不全面也不正确。患者如果通过阅读网上知识（自学成才），来影响医生的专业抉择，这样就走偏了。比如有些患者在网上看到很多"微创"治疗的好处，但是实际上并不真正明了这个"微创"的方法和含义，大部分以为"用简单轻微的处理就能达到传统手术的效果"，所以有的上来就问能不能"微创"做，如果不能就到其他地方去做。这实际上大大地影响了医生的专业决定，因为有些肿瘤手术腹腔镜可以做得非常好（如妇科手术），而有些病情却是开腹手术能够达到更好的疗效，也许更加"微小创伤"；还有些医院腹腔镜开展不那么广泛，却在患者"执念"下强行开展，常常效果不佳。用什么方法治疗和手术，这些本该是医务人员根据专业判断作出的决定，有时却受到了患者和家属的影响。

另一方面，不少患者反映，一些医院的医生直接让患者自行选择治疗方案：可以手术或者用药，你们自己来选吧。患者会一头雾水，他们也不懂医，如何自己选择治疗方案？但是医务人员可能经历另一种不良体验，就是当他们为患者决定治疗方案后，如果引起不良治疗后果，会被指责甚至承担责任。如果这样的话，还不如一开始就让你自己来定，这样后果都是你自己承担了。这个现象并不正常，但是存在。这个社会在短短一代人里面经历了太快的发展、太多的动荡和变迁，有些人心浮气躁、急切，还带来很多相互不信任感；人的受教育程度和文明层次也存在很大的差异，所以患者和家属到底要多深地介入医疗决断，很难把握。

在中国传统人文精神下，有些恶性、病情严重的病症还不能让患者直接知道（这个和西方正好相反），所以当患者和家属参与决策时，会增加困难程度。比如既要说服患者接受手术治疗，又不能和患者明说这是一个恶性病变，不切除可能短期内危及生命。

所以如何把握患者和家属在专业医疗决断中的参与程度是一个有意义的话题，也可能是一个永远在路上的问题，因为随着时代的发展、文明的提高，患者在医疗决策中的参与程度和医患关系本身都会不断地变化和调整，我们可能会在不同阶段一直讨论这个话题。本次我们请到了浙江大学医学院的徐骁教授，请他来对这个问题进行分析探讨，他很有想法希望能引起大家的重视和讨论。

医疗决策的难题：患方是否适宜参与？

周军彬[1, 2, 3]　徐　骁[1, 2, 3]

[1]浙江大学医学院
[2]浙江省肿瘤与智能医学整合重点实验室
[3]浙江大学器官移植研究所

医者从来便是一个神圣的职业。对仁人志士而言，"不为良相，便为良医"，医者寄托了他们美好的憧憬；对寻常百姓而言，"杏林春满，妙手回春"，他们不吝用最美好的词汇赞美医者。人们往往将治疗的成功都归因于医者的医术高明，却往往忽略了患方在医疗决策中的作用。随着全民教育和健康水平的提升，患方对参与医疗决策的意愿不断增强。我们不禁思考：医疗决策作为一项专业性极强的医学活动，是否应该让相对"外行"的患方参与进来？如何参与才能为患者带来更好的临床获益？

因病制宜：患方参与医疗决策不能一概而论

我们必须承认的是：在现有医疗环境中，受制于医疗资源有限等客观因素，让患方全面参与医疗决策是不现实的，因为这势必会拖慢医疗节奏，甚至贻误治疗时机，可能对患者个人生命健康和社会整体医疗保障产生不利；但将患方完全排斥在医疗决策之外也显然有悖医学发展进程。

就目前而言，医疗决策模式不应一概而论，而要"因病制宜"，根据疾病的性质来决定患方在医疗决策中的参与程度。

在我们近年来开展的肝胆胰疑难病多学科诊疗（multi-disciplinary treatment，MDT）中，患方是全程参与的。实践证明，就疑难病例而言，鼓励患方参与医疗决策并不会产生明显负面影响，反而对提高医患沟通效率、构建和谐医患关系有所裨益，也有助于提升患者对治疗方案的依从性。

以终末期肝病为例，肝移植是目前唯一根治手段，患方既对此抱有很大期待，也往往心存疑虑。虽然肝移植技术目前已较为成熟，但仍存在一定风险，且术后多需要长期随访治疗。因此，以患者临床获益为导向，我们会在术前通过MDT等方式与患方充分沟通，使其对疾病本质和手术预后形成正确认知与合理期望，并在此基础上共同制定个体化诊疗方案。这有助于患方更清晰地理解肝移植手术的获益与风险，在心理上更容易接受并配合治疗。

临床上还有部分患者因肝源紧缺等因素需行亲体肝移植。在这种情况下，供者是与患者利益相关的特殊群体，其作为健康人接受器官捐献手术，在身心上要经受重大考验；同时，医方也面临来自供、受者双方的压力和复杂的伦理问题，在手术的推进上可能遭遇诸多困难。以哥哥（健康人）给弟弟（终末期肝病患者）捐献部分肝脏为例，此时，哥哥及其亲属（如妻子等）也应纳入医疗决策流程，并鼓励他们充分表达期望值和价值观，结合其经济、文化、宗教、家庭、年龄以及弟弟病情等因素综合考量，最终决定是否捐献以及确定最佳移植方案。供、受者双方共同参与医疗决策，有助于其在充分理解手术获益与风险的基础上达成共识；另外，移植医生要连续实施两台性命攸关的手术，承受着巨大压力，患方的理解与支持可以给予我们更多信心。

以上，对于疑难病例，我们通过积极寻求患方参与医疗决策，在不违背医学诊疗规范的前提下尽可能满足患方意愿，是对其生命权和健康权的最大尊重。而对于部分常见病和多发病而言，例如胆囊炎等良性疾病，相应的治疗方案往往已十分成熟，且一般能获得较好治疗效果；对于此类患者，则可在常规知情同意的基础上，由医方主导诊疗方案的制定与执行，而无须过度强调患方对医疗决策的参与，这也能避免其因此而产生无谓的疑虑。

"主导权"与"参与权"：医患双方权利的博弈

"医非博不能通，非通不能精，非精不能专"，医疗决策作为一项专业性极强的医学活动，需要以长期医学积累和大量临床实践为基础。显然，多数患方作为非医学人士，无论在知识还是实践方面，都很难达到医疗决策所要求的水平。因此，我们要把握好患方在医疗决策中参与的"度"，过分强调患方的参与可能会使医疗活动走向另一个极端。

随着近年来互联网的飞速发展，医患矛盾被无限放大，部分患方容易受不良报道影响而对医务人员产生误解，他们宁愿相信自己在网络上查来的信息，也不愿相信医生仔细评估后给出的诊疗意见，甚至"要求"医生按照自己的想法来治疗。我们可以理解这部分患方因缺乏信任而做出的不合理行为，但这往往令我们在规范诊治上处处掣肘、举步维艰。

从另一方面来说，若医方一味迎合患方不合理的要求而丧失主见，甚至在患方"影响"下施以不符合医学规范的治疗，那恰恰是对患者生命权和健康权不负责任的表现，也是对其自身职业价值观和医学精神的违背。若医方丧失了对诊疗过程的主导权，就像汽车司机将方向盘交给没有驾驶资质的乘客，对医患双方均有弊无利，但受害更大的终究是患方。

医疗决策中医患双方权利的僭越会加剧矛盾激化，因此，我们有必要认真界定"主导权"与"参与权"这两项权利在医疗决策中的内涵与归属。医疗决策是专业而严肃的医学活动，其"主导权"理应归属于医方，即医方在充分了解病情后，依据相关诊疗指南和临床经验针对患者制定个体化诊疗方案；而患方则具有对医疗决策的"参与权"，即将自身信息如实告知医生后获得相应反馈，并对给出的治疗方案作出最终选择。医方与患方应在医疗决策中各司其职、互相尊重，患方不能随意干预医疗方案的制定，而医方也不能剥夺患方知情与选择的权利。

与时俱进：人工智能时代医疗决策新模式探索

事实上，我们并不排斥患方参与医疗决策，因为这有助于提升其对医疗服务的满意度并促进医患关系的和谐发展，何乐而不为？但我们在临床实践中也经常碰到这样的情景：部分患方以"不懂"为由不愿参与医疗决策，甚至不愿承担任何医疗后果，还有部分患方虽然"不懂"却硬要对成熟的治疗方案"瞎指挥"，让我们哭笑不得。患方医学知识的匮乏是造成这一尴尬局面的重要原因，如何打破医患之间疾病知识不对等的信息壁垒成为问题关键。

令人欣喜的是，近年来人工智能技术的飞速发展让我们看到了解决这个老大难问题的曙光。例如近来爆火的聊天机器人程序ChatGPT引发了媒体热议，我们是否能借助此类工具来寻求医患间疾病知识在一定程度上的"对等"呢？ChatGPT毕竟不是专业的医学工具，其给出的疾病知识的准确性和时效性仍有待时间检验。但事实上医学界早已有人着手开发此类工具，一类是面向医生的临床决策支持工具（clinical decision support system，CDSS），另一类是面向患者的决策辅助工具（patient decision aids，PDA）。这些工具旨在促进医患之间信息高效互通和患方对疾病知识的获取。已有研究表明这些工具的使用对于提升医疗质量、患者依从性和服务满意度有积极作用。

医疗决策工具有望消弭医患间疾病知识的鸿沟，使患方以更"专业"的姿态参与医疗决策。但考虑到医学学科的严肃性与医学知识的快速更新，此类工具的大规模推广应用仍需要更多的实践检验并持续优化。尤其是在国内相关研究起步较晚的环境下，距离真正实现医疗决策工具"入户到家"仍有一段较长的路。

结语：共建和谐医患命运共同体

人类文明与医学发展具有前进性，让患方更多地参与医疗决策是大势所趋。我们应当意识到，面对疾病，医患从来都是同心一体，积极鼓励与引导患方参与医疗决策，是医学人文精神和职业价值观的重要体现，更是新时期患方对我们提出的更高要求。医患双方要充分厘清自己在医疗决策中的权利边界，互相尊重与合作，而不是互相僭越与猜疑。但就目前而言，我们尚不具备全面实行"医患共同决策"的必要条件，还需要相关政策和法律的支持、医疗服务机构的倡导、医务人员的积极响应、患方的共同参与以及专业工具的辅助。医疗决策模式的变革是新时期构建和谐医患命运共同体的需要，要求我们医疗相关行业所有从业者和参与者共同努力。

参考文献

［1］ China Youth Daily. Experiment on doctor-patient relationship by three academicians. Available online: http://zqb.cyol.com/html/2015-06/24/nw.D110000zgqnb_20150624_1-12.htm

［2］ Ling S, Jiang G, Que Q, et al. Liver transplantation in patients with liver failure: Twenty years of experience from China. Liver Int 2022; 42: 2110-6.

［3］ Gallaher JR, Charles A. Acute Cholecystitis: A Review. JAMA 2022; 327: 965-75.

［4］ Agoritsas T, Heen AF, Brandt L, et al. Decision aids that really promote shared decision making: the pace quickens. BMJ 2015; 350: g7624.

［5］ Graber ML. Reaching 95%: decision support tools are the surest way to improve diagnosis now. BMJ Qual Saf 2022; 31: 415-8.

［6］ Yu SF, Wang YY, Deng T, et al. Medical decision-making series 1: development of shared decision-making at home and abroad. Med Recapitulate 2020; 30: 159-67.

The difficulty of medical decision-making: should patients be involved?

Zhou Junbin[1,2,3], Xu Xiao[1,2,3]

[1]Zhejiang University School of Medicine, Hangzhou, China
[2]Key Laboratory of Integrated Oncology and Intelligent Medicine of Zhejiang Province, Hangzhou, China
[3]Institute of Organ Transplantation, Zhejiang University, Hangzhou, China

Keywords: Communication; decision making; patient participation; physician-patient relations

Introduction

The success or failure of treatment has long been attributed to the doctors alone, but the role of patients in the medical decision-making (MDM) process has often been ignored. As medical development and health needs increase, the desire of patients to participate in MDM continues to grow. This raises the question: should patients be involved in such a highly professional medical activity? How can their involvement bring better clinical benefits?

Tailor-made approaches for different disease cases: patient involvement in MDM should not be generalized

We must acknowledge that in the current healthcare environment, it is unrealistic to fully involve patients in MDM due to objective conditions such as limited medical resources. Such involvement could inevitably slow down the pace of medical treatment and threaten timely treatment in some acute diseases. However, exclusion of patients from MDM is contrary to the course of medical development [1] Currently, our MDM model should not be generalized but tailored to different cases, with the degree of patient involvement determined based on the nature of the disease.

In our multidisciplinary treatment (MDT) for difficult hepatobiliary and pancreatic diseases, patients are involved throughout the process. We have found that encouraging patients to participate in MDM in difficult cases could help to improve the efficiency of doctor-patient communication, the patients' trust in the medical team, and their compliance with treatment plans.

Taking end-stage liver disease as an example, liver transplantation (LT) is currently the only curative treatment [2]. Patients have high expectations for this treatment as well as doubts and concerns. Although LT is relatively mature, there are still risks involved, and long-term postoperative management is required. Therefore, we always communicate with patients before LT through MDT and other methods to help them form a correct understanding of the disease and the surgical plan. We jointly develop personalized treatment plans with patients, and that helps them better understand the benefits and risks of the surgery, which makes it easier for patients to make decisions and cooperate with the transplant team.

In clinical practice, there are some patients who need to receive living donor LT. In this scenario, the donor is a healthy person receiving organ donation surgery, which presents great physical and psychological challenge; at the same time, the doctors face pressure from both the donor and the recipient, and may encounter difficulties in moving forward with the surgery. In the case of an older brother donating part of his liver to his younger brother, the older brother and his relatives (such as his wife) should also be included in the MDM, encouraged to fully express their expectations and preferences, and to take into account their financial,

守在生命的边缘
医者沉思录

cultural, religious, family, age and the disease condition, in order to decide whether to donate and to determine the best surgery plan. The joint participation of both donors and recipients in MDM helps them to reach a consensus based on a full understanding of the benefits and risks of the surgery; on the other hand, the understanding and support of the patient can give transplant surgeons more confidence.

For difficult cases, we actively seek the patient's involvement in MDM to the extent possible without violating medical treatment standards, in order to give the greatest respect to their right to life and health. However, for some common or frequently occurring diseases, such as benign conditions like cholecystitis, the corresponding treatment protocols are often well established and can generally achieve good results [3]. For these patients, MDM can be led by the doctors based on routine informed consent, without overemphasizing the involvement of patients, which can also avoid their unnecessary doubts.

The game of rights between doctors and patients: the right to lead vs. the right to participate

MDM is a highly specialized medical activity. However, most patients do not have the same level of medical knowledge and clinical experience as doctors. Therefore, we must determine the extent to which patients participate in MDM. Overemphasizing patients' participation may lead to unexpected outcomes.

The unrestricted development of the internet has amplified medical disputes, as some patients are easily influenced by negative reports and thus misunderstand doctors, preferring to trust the information they find on the internet rather than professional suggestions from doctors, and may even "demand" doctors to treat them according to their own ideas. While we can understand to some extent the unreasonable behavior of these patients, it often undermines standardized care and may result in poor prognosis.

On the other hand, if the doctor caters to the unreasonable demands of the patient and lose their initiative, even under the "influence" of the patient to administer treatment that is not in line with medical norms, it is actually an irresponsible behavior that violates the patient's right to life and health, as well as a violation of their own professional values and medical spirit.

The arrogation of rights between doctors and patients can lead to undesirable outcomes and exacerbate their conflicts. Therefore, it is necessary to carefully define the attribution of the "right to lead" and "the right to participate" between doctors and patients. MDM, as a professional medical activity, should be dominated by doctors, meaning that they are primary responsible for the development of treatment plan, while the patients have the right to participate, that is, after informing the doctors of their condition, they should receive feedback and make the final choice for the treatment plan given. Doctors and patients each have a role and should respect each other's rights in MDM.

Keeping up with the times: exploring new models of MDM in the age of artificial intelligence

In fact, we encourage patients to participate in MDM, as it helps to improve their satisfaction with medical services and promotes a harmonious doctor-patient relationship. However, in clinical practice, we often encounter situations where some patients are unwilling to participate in MDM on the grounds that they do not understand medicine or do not want to bear the medical consequences. On the contrary, some patients who lack medical knowledge insist on "commanding" better treatments, which leaves doctors helpless. The unequal distribution of medical knowledge between doctors and patients creates information barriers that need to be broken down.

Fortunately, rapidly evolving artificial intelligence provides us with hope to solve the above problem. One promising example that has garnered public attention is the chatbot program ChatGPT. It is important to note that ChatGPT is not a professional tool and the accuracy and timeliness of its medical knowledge still need to be improved. However, the medical community has long been working on developing such tools, including clinical decision support systems (CDSS) designed for doctors and patient decision aids (PDA) designed for patients. These tools aim to promote efficient information exchange between doctors and patients and help patients acquire disease knowledge. Studies have shown that these tools are effective in improving medical quality, patient compliance, and service satisfaction [4,5].

These tools are expected to bridge the gap in disease knowledge between doctors and patients, empowering patients to participate in MDM in a more informed manner. However, due to the gravity of the medical discipline and the constant updates in medical knowledge, the widespread implementation and application of such tools require further practical testing and continuous optimization. Especially in China, where related research started relatively late, there is still a long way to go before these tools can truly become commonplace.

Conclusion: building a harmonious community of shared destiny between doctors and patients

With the continuous development of human civilization and medicine, there is a trend toward greater patients' participation in MDM. We should realize that doctors and patients are always on the same side in the face of diseases. Encouraging and guiding patients to be more involved in MDM is not only a reflection of medical humanism and professional values, but also a higher demand from patients in this era. To make this work, doctors and patients must clearly define their rights and responsibilities in MDM and work together with mutual respect and cooperation. However, despite the trend toward shared decision-making, we still lack the necessary conditions to fully implement this approach. It will require the support of relevant policies and laws, the advocacy of medical institutions, the positive response of doctors, the participation of patients, and the assistance of professional tools [6]. Transforming MDM models is essential to create a harmonious doctor-patient community of shared destiny in this new era, which require the joint efforts of all medical professionals and participants in our medical-related industry.

References

[1] China Youth Daily. Experiment on doctor-patient relationship by three academicians. Available online: http://zqb.cyol.com/html/2015-06/24/nw.D110000zgqnb_20150624_1-12.htm

[2] Ling S, Jiang G, Que Q, et al. Liver transplantation in patients with liver failure: Twenty years of experience from China. Liver Int 2022; 42: 2110-6.

[3] Gallaher JR, Charles A. Acute Cholecystitis: A Review. JAMA 2022; 327: 965-75.

[4] Agoritsas T, Heen AF, Brandt L, et al. Decision aids that really promote shared decision making: the pace quickens. BMJ 2015; 350: g7624.

[5] Graber ML. Reaching 95%: decision support tools are the surest way to improve diagnosis now. BMJ Qual Saf 2022; 31: 415-8.

[6] Yu SF, Wang YY, Deng T, et al. Medical decision-making series 1: development of shared decision-making at home and abroad. Med Recapitulate 2020; 30: 159-67.

主编导读（六）

关于"临终关怀"，这篇文章可能改变你的认知

临终关怀：急需建立和完善的体系。

我的很多患者都是肿瘤晚期患者。这些晚期患者，虽然已经没有有效治疗方案了，但他们还是需要良好和温馨的照顾，但是目前的医疗体系里显然短缺了这部分业务。

临床医生常常能体会到一种尴尬，我们多年的老患者，有些已经慢慢成为老朋友，但是当他们到了疾病最后一期的时候，似乎没有一个合适的地方能安排他们继续维持。各级繁忙的医院一般不愿意收治这类患者，因为这是无法完成的肿瘤治疗任务，却可能占用本不充裕的床位和医务人员的精力，这些床位一般会留给需要通过手术和药物治疗的患者。这也是合理的。但是每当看到这些晚期的老患者们面临这种情况时一脸踌躇、无助和失落的神态，我心里还是很难受的。但之后大凡都被继续接诊的新患者带来的繁忙而自然淡化了。

实际上终末期的患者自己也知道，就疾病本身而言，到了这个阶段也应该没有转机了。他们需要的是一个能被良好安置、被悉心照顾的地方。在那里他们可以被解除疼痛及其他症状，做一些必要的支持治疗。人是需要有一个安心和安身之处的，但是在目前的医疗体系中找到这么一个地方还是比较困难的。虽然我们已经看到了一些正在进行的努力（如合作建立安宁医疗病房等），但是大部分患者最后是通过自己或家人自行联系，不规则地分散到各处地段或者基层医院里，实际上是一种无奈。

在西方，医疗体系里有一套临终关怀系统，已经行之有效地运行了很多年。他们各国有各国的特点，应该是根据自己的国情演变、完善而成的。这些理念和做法是值得我们学习的。虽然可能不能完全照搬（东方人的家庭、亲戚关系不一样），但是有很多理念和构架很值得我们借鉴。近年来，虽然中国国力增强，但是我们不能意气

用事，还是应该学习西方很多优秀的、成熟的系统和做法。

　　奇怪的是，当我回忆起30多年前我刚刚行医的年代里，好像医患双方都感受不到患者在疾病晚期时有强烈的临终关怀需求。那个时候一旦患者病入膏肓，家属就会自己将患者拉回去，之后怎么处理，也不甚了解。那为什么现在这个问题慢慢凸显出来成为一个迫切需求了呢？我觉得还是生活水平和社会文明发展的关系。在温饱还没有解决或需要花很大努力去解决的时代里，有很多人文的细节容易被忽略或遮盖起来，显得不那么突出。如我小时候随意将一块写有"小偷"的牌子挂在胡同里被逮住的小偷的脖子上，在玩耍时残害小动物也没感到愧疚等，这些行为放在现在就完全不可想象了。现在的年轻人明显比以前的我们文明得多，他们以后还会构建一个更美好、更合理、更温暖的社会体系，带着旧思想的老人终会退出。所以从这个变化上来看，晚期患者需要尊严地活完最后一段时间的需求将会越来越强烈，他们应该在人生最后一刻活在有尊严、有温情、相对舒适的环境里，这个漏缺我们要赶紧补上。

该关注我国的临终关怀了

丛亚丽

北京大学医学人文学院　医学伦理与法律系
《柳叶刀》死亡的价值委员会委员

临终关怀：需要关注的大问题

本以为对死亡的问题有了理解，直至加入《柳叶刀》死亡的价值委员会，才发现原来的理解尚浅；本以为对临终关怀也有所了解，当被询问"每当我的老病患经过了手术、复发、再治疗、再扩散的姑息治疗以后，没有办法继续在北京协和医院这种医院里为他服务了，因为这种病情已经无法在我们这里接受住院治疗了。然后那个时候，老病患会问我，那还有什么地方能够去吗？……"我才发现自己对此问题的感受是多么苍白。也促成对此问题的一点思考。

其实，从我们自己的患者没有地方得到临终照护，可以得知，偌大的中国，绝大部分临终患者没有其容身之处；从我们医生自己所在的医院无法继续帮助生命末期的患者，可以知道，无论是综合医院还是专科医院，可以提供安宁疗护的医院，是多么有限；从我们医生看到患者的处境，而想到自己未来可能遭遇的情境，那么，所有的医生也面临相似的未来，而我们每个人都将迎来那么一天。

临终关怀溯源

英国的Dame Cicely Saunders早在1948年便开始涉足对临终者的照顾，这与其宗教情怀相关。她先后作为护士、社会工作者和医生的角色接受培训，并率先把照顾临终者的理念和实践带到现实中。其背景因素包括从20世纪50年代开始出现的大部分人是死在医院中，而非自己家中的现象，这个变化促使了医院必须提供大量的治疗和帮助去帮助患者延续生命，但也意味着医疗行业逐渐把死亡这一结局看作医学的失败。

针对这种情况，Saunders创办了医院St Christopher's，1967年7月24日医院正式对外开放。Saunders 2005年7月14日卒于伦敦，欣慰的是，临终前她在自己创办的临终关怀医院接受过一段时间的照护。

人们一般用身心社灵（身体—心理—社会—灵性）来说明临终关怀的内涵。St Christopher's医院这样界定临终关怀：对患者从生理、精神和心理完好方面进行整体的照护路径，它不仅是对临终者的照护，而且在医疗实践整合方面也标志着一个新开端。

现在的圣·克里斯托弗医院与时俱进，不仅为住院的患者提供多种形式的服务，也为其所在的社区提供相关服务，包括为居家的患者和家庭提供帮助、提供线上服务和线上活动等。

临终关怀的现状

各国的患者在临终阶段对于疼痛的管理，是衡量死亡质量和死亡是否平等的一个重要评价指标。从全球范围看，有人能享受到临终照护，有人享受不到；有的人希望得到临终照护但却享受不起；有的人能享受得起但又不接纳。其中的差异，有些是观念的原因，有些是制度的原因。

《柳叶刀》就安宁疗护也曾组建委员会，安宁疗护委员会在2018年发布了题为《缓解姑息治疗和疼痛舒缓的可及性深渊——全民健康覆盖的必要条件》的报告。报告提到，全球范围内的临终关怀现状的特点之一表现为发达国家和发展中国家之间的鲜明对比，以及贫穷人群对安宁疗护的不可及问题。实质就是死亡不平等的现实，死亡不平等还是个较新的概念，其中主要体现在临终阶段。

我国的伴随疼痛的临终患者人数多，但在疼痛缓解药品的消费量却不多。参照十年前的数据，美国患者人均使用68 000mg疼痛缓解药品，而中国患者人均使用量则为314mg，仅满足不到16%的患者。其中既有对疼痛忍受的理念的原因，也有医疗系列内部的理念的转变得不彻底等原因，而导致一些临终患者遭受了极大的折磨。临终关怀问题，不仅是关涉每个人的问题，也是社会生活质量提升的一个关键指标。但这个问题并没有引起应有的关注。

从反思医生和医学的角色开始

文章开头提到的现状可以归纳为这几个担忧。

首先，患者怕自己没有尊严地活着，怕没有地方得到照顾，没有地方安心地死去。

其次，家庭作为临终者主要的照护场所，因缺乏社会支持和必要的资源而不堪重负，即便自己尽力了却不确定患者是否满意，也担心周围对自己的负面评价。

最后，医生既担心自己的老病患没有地方被照顾，也担心自己那个时候该怎么办。

可以说，面对这些困境的包括医生在内的所有人。

我们与临终的关系不健康：医生/医学难辞其咎。

死亡价值委员会官网上的第一个图片和一段话，便鲜明地点出来：现代医疗系统与死亡之间的关系不健康，我们正在努力使其更健康（图1）。

Modern health care has an unhealthy relationship with death. We are exploring how to make it healthier.

图1 与死亡的不健康关系

我们都非常熟悉的"知识就是力量"的提出者Francis Bacon早在16世纪末便把医学的职能分成维护健康、治疗疾病和延长寿命三类。随着现代医学的发展，医生的职责逐渐被定位在了第三个方面。逐渐地，人们生活的方方面面都需要制度化医疗系统的干涉。医学是规则的制定者，医生是死亡判定的仲裁者，人只能死在医院中。

只有医生经过努力后没有能力制止死亡时，才宣布死亡。这时，这个人才能死。

不难看出，造成这种不健康关系的原因之一，就是我们现代医学，包括我们医生，是我们自己把自己塑造成与死神作斗争和不接纳死亡的角色。或者说，是我们医疗系统自己把我们与临终和死亡的关系弄僵了。

探索临终关怀之路，医疗系统当仁不让

安宁疗护之花正在喀拉拉邦盛开

喀拉拉邦（Kerala）是印度西南部的一个很小的邦，拥有3500万人口，然而在全球却是安宁疗护做得最好的地方，真正做到了将低费用、公平可及、共同参与，以及大批量培训社会工作者等融合在其中。

其成功的原因可以归结为针对如何看待疾病、临终、照护和哀伤等的理念和一系列范式的转变。起初是由两名医生 M R Rajagopal（死亡的价值委员会成员）和 Suresh Kumar 以及一名志愿者 Asoka Kumar 在1993年成立的一个民间组织。初始目的是管理重病患者的疼痛和其他症状，工作地点是门诊，尽管社区捐款支持这项工作并有志愿者协助，但该项目是基于姑息治疗的临床模型。

随后这种模式的缺陷很快显现，因为很多家庭没有能力把患者送到诊所，否则将失去一天的工资，难以维持生计；另外，患者的精神和照顾需求在诊所难以被满足。后来便改革，发展成志愿者去家里探望和帮助家人照顾他们。随后的范式转变为集中在医务人员和社会民众对临终和照护的态度和理念上，提倡所有初级卫生保健中心嵌入这种以家庭为基础、由志愿者主导的临终关怀模式，并应纳入全民健康覆盖的核心组成部分。

通过印度最大的地区性报纸开展媒体宣传活动，向公众讲述临终或患有慢性病的人们的需求……该报在三天内接到了5000多个希望在活动中做志愿者的电话。一个志愿者的"我们看到了煎熬而不

是疾病"点出了临终照护需要更多的社会支持，需要更多的资源进入卫生保健领域。第二次转变迅速扩大了可用和可重新整合的服务数量，并将其融入主流医疗保健服务的体系中。这一年，是2005年。

喀拉拉邦地区政府响应社区行动的热潮，制定了相应的姑息治疗政策。

该政策于2008年宣布，指出姑息治疗应该是参与性的，并与社区参与者密切合作。它进一步描述了所有初级卫生保健单位应如何与当地志愿者单位合作提供姑息治疗。于是在印度的2000家姑息治疗服务机构中，80%位于喀拉拉邦，并培训了数万名志愿者，出现了现实的乌托邦。至少在喀拉拉邦的每个地区都能提供尽管有限但却被估计覆盖超过70%的有需要的人的姑息治疗服务。

喀拉拉邦的安宁疗护，给我们展示了"桃花源"式的临终者照护模式。它成功的经验可以归结为：有远见的医生发起、受益于当地的社区自治和大量志愿者参与的传统、对当地文化传统模式的尊重和密切合作，促使建成了死亡与慢性病的社区网络；最后也离不开当地的卫生政策改革，使得阿片类药物应用于临终者在现实中可及。

死亡的价值委员会提出的建议包括承认并认可死亡的价值，把死亡日常化，鼓励分享死亡叙事，完善相关人际网络，纳入患者家属、更广泛的社区成员以及专业人员，以引导对临终者、照护者和哀伤者的支持等，其实有受到喀拉拉邦经验的启发。

临终关怀的根本出路——从观念到制度的转变

活着和死着是人的生命的一体两面，这是每个人都需要的生命哲学

一个人走到生命的最后阶段已经很脆弱了。我们常人正值壮年时都难以忍受的痛苦，临终者如何能耐受？人们多认为，死亡是我们要极力避免的，死亡能逃避，但疼痛不能逃避，为此，当然要忍受痛苦。一方面，我们在生理和躯体层面，被灌输忍受疼痛的折磨；另一方面，却在精神层面鼓励人们要克服对死亡的恐惧。如果生理

关过不了，心理关更难了。这样的理念和程序，存在难以落实的悖论。

中国关于死亡观念的历史文献很多，简要地说，除了佛教，我们对于死亡，多是逃避的态度。有的也多体现在探究人生的意义，死亡本身没有什么意义，死了就意味着可以休息了，而活着不能休息，得奋斗。西方哲学史中有较多对死亡的探讨，其中德国的哲学家海德格尔最为著名，大家熟悉的"向死而生"便是他的智慧。他认为，正因为有了死亡，你才成为你，但若不把死亡考虑进生活之中，终究还是把死亡和生活割裂开。

海德格尔的"向死而生"，是说活着和死着，是生活的两个时间向度，是生命本质含义的一体两面。我们活着，是在实践生命；但我们也应该知道，人从出生便在走向死亡，因此自己同时也在死着，关于死亡的思考其实是每个人都与生俱来的生命哲学。而临终，是把这个一体两面同时呈现在我们面前，具有强大的冲击力。

临终和死亡是生活的一部分，并不难理解，只是多数人不会把二者切实地看为一体两面，潜意识中不去触碰死亡那一面，也自然不会延伸到临终关怀。桑德斯的"因为你是你，所以你很重要；我们在乎你，直到生命的最后一刻"。

死亡是临终者送给我们人类的礼物

把临终、死亡和礼物联系起来，是受《死亡的价值报告》内容的启发。其中提到马塞尔·莫斯和列维纳斯关于礼物与死亡的关系。莫斯的《礼物》一书提到"礼物的灵魂"，是说人们对它既期待又敬畏，又不敢独自占有。接受礼物便意味着有了不得不回礼的义务，否则这个精灵将会破坏自己的生活。

送礼物，接受礼物和回礼，即给予、接受和回报，被看作三种义务。有尊严地回报是一种强制性的义务。如果不做回报，或者没有毁坏相等价值的东西，那将会丢一辈子的脸。拒绝收礼物，就表明害怕回报。

他人的死亡，让我们对生命有很多思考，这是临终者给照护他的人和周围人的一个礼物，我们每个人都曾经或即将接收到这份礼物。如果我们能真正认识到死亡是临终者给我们人类的礼物，我们就要回报临终者，把对于临终者个体的照护在卫生制度中予以体现，而不是某个家庭的个体行为，这样每个人都会在生命的最后阶段得到应有的照顾和关怀，解除身心的痛苦，提高死亡质量，促进死亡平等。

把死亡看作礼物，虽然这不是我们熟悉的观点，但从前述的分析可以看出它的历史逻辑和未来前景。我们文化非常崇尚礼尚往来，而且民间还有还愿的做法。我们可以探讨这个理念如何能帮助我们转变理念，从理念到实践上实现对临终者的照护。

医生的角色：从我们做起

现代医学的飞速发展挽救了无数生命，大大减少了患者的痛苦，但也使我们迷失了医学的目的。我们以为在技术的帮助下可以无所不能，而不自觉地不惜一切代价维系生命，医生认为所有的精力都应该用在抢救、抢救、抢救上，理念中还没有充分留出照护临终患者的空间。

但当临终来临，患者正在承受煎熬，那么让医学发挥奇迹的理念该让位于临终患者关怀了。即便有医生持有临终关怀的理念，但医疗系统和多数医生也被社会和患者家属裹挟着，被要求疲于奔命地救治患者。

2017年，北京市、上海市、吉林省、河南省、四川省等地参照世界卫生组织的标准，启动了第一批安宁疗护试点；2019年5月，全国第二批启动了71个试点。但现实中还有许多障碍没有解决。例如，有些服务支出没有定价，不允许收费，只能自己想办法，或者请志愿者帮助等——这是安宁疗护专业人员普遍表述的工作困难。

笔者认为，我国目前安宁疗护发展的最大瓶颈还是在于观念，不仅是政策制定者的观念，还包括患者及其家属的观念。很多患者因不接受临终，也就是他不接受死亡，而失去临终关怀的机会；或者因家属不接受而使得患者无法享受相关服务。其次，安宁疗护面临的是能力提升的瓶颈，不仅是缺乏有安宁疗护胜任能力的医务人员，还包括我们尚需更好的医疗机构层面的医疗资源配置。

现实中已有一些针对在乡村开展临终关怀的实践探讨，提出提升村医介入临终关怀的条件和能力以及充分利用民间资源助力村医介入乡村临终关怀的对策。英国的利物浦照护路径（liverpool care pathway）研究也给我们以启示，即把临终照护模式应用在大医院或急救中心会以失败而告终。此研究得出的教训主要在于医生缺乏培训，尤其关键的是医生群体关于临终关怀的理念不足。结论是，不是大医院不能提供临终关怀服务，而是缺乏培训；医院目前使用新技术的方法不适宜，传统的任务清单的勾选模式的做法也不适合临终关怀，而是应该用脑用心体会患者的需求。

为满足我国大量的需要照护的临终者需求，除了专业的安宁疗护试点医院，重担仍然落在我们每个医生和每家医院肩上。因为这是基于临终患者的需求，只要有需求，就应有相应的照护在场——无论他处在哪个类型的医院。我国正在建立的安宁疗护体系，如果能吸取已有的经验教训，充分挖掘死亡作为礼物带给我们的行为动力，那么我国的临终关怀有望成为消解我们民众死亡焦虑的一种理念、一种模式，甚至是一种文化。

对此，整个社会的理念需要转变，因为临终关怀绝不只是医疗系统内部的事情，喀拉拉邦的经历已经告诉我们，一个社会要转变观念，需要有个群体带领大家率先走出第一步。虽然全社会在多个层面面临处理与临终之间关系的挑战，但把握好这个尺度，只有医生有能力作专业判断。医疗系统和医生群体作为临终关怀的引领者，应当仁不让。

参考文献

［1］Illich I. Limits to Medicine: Medical Nemesis, the Expropriation of Health. London: Marion Boyars Publishers; 2013: 190, 205.

［2］Institute for Advanced Study of the Americas. Lancet Commission on Palliative

Care and Pain Relief. Background Resources. SHS and DOME by Country. 2018. Available online: https://mia.as.miami.edu/_ assets/pdf/SHS%20and%20 DOME%20by%20 Country_20180410.pdf

[3] Knaul FM, Farmer PE, Krakauer EL, et al. Alleviating the access abyss in palliative care and pain relief-an imperative of universal health coverage: the Lancet Commission Report. Lancet 2018; 391: 1391-454. Erratum in: Lancet 2018; 391: 2212.

[4] Mauss M. The Gifts. Translated by Ji Z. Shanghai: Shanghai People's Publishing House; 2002: 70-4.

[5] Sallnow L, Smith R, Ahmedzai SH, et al. Report of the Lancet Commission on the Value of Death: bringing death back into life. Lancet 2022; 399: 837-84.

Difficulties and opportunities of hospice care —the role of doctors

Cong Yali

Department of Medical Ethics and Law, the School of Health Humanities, Peking University, Beijing, China

Unhealthy relationship with death

Our relationship with death is unhealthy, as the Lancet Commission on the Value of Death website pointed out clearly on their home page: "Modern health care has an unhealthy relationship with death. We are exploring how to make it healthier." (*Figure 1*).

As early as the end of the 16th century, Francis Bacon divided medicine into three offices: preservation of health, the cure of disease, and prolongation of life. With the development of modern medicine, the responsibility of doctors has gradually been set on the third. For this, Ivan Illich sharply criticized that, the relationship between death and life was natural before, but today, such a relationship has been largely distorted. Death becomes a commodity and the socialized medicine becomes a tool of the so-called "the managed life", medicine is the rule maker, doctors are the umpire of death. The rules forbid leaving the game and dying in any fashion that has not been specified by the umpire. Death no longer occurs except as the self-fulfilling prophecy of the medicine man [1].

It is hard for modern health care to find excuses from such unhealthy situation. It is we ourselves who portray ourselves as fighters who are against death and refuse to accept the arrival of death.

Hospice care: death inequality from a global perspective

The unhealthy relationship with death is primarily manifested in the end-of-life stage.

According to the data in *Table 1* [2], from 2011 to 2013, the number of terminally ill patients in China who suffered from pain is 17 times that of the UK, but the consumption of pain relief medicine in China is less than half that of the UK, and the US is 50 times that of China. Hospice care globally shows a stark contrast between developed and developing countries, as well as the inaccessibility of the poor to palliative care [3]. Pain control of patients at the end of life in various countries is an important parameter to measure the quality of death and the equality of death. From a global perspective, some people have access to hospice care, while others don't; some people hope to get hospice care but cannot afford it; some people can afford it but refuse to accept it. Such discrepancies are due to individual values differences, but more relates to the inequality of death caused by society and system.

The fundamental path of hospice care development—the transformation of concepts

Living and dying are two sides of our human life

Some cultures feel comfortable talking about death, while others prefer to purposefully neglect this subject. Chinese culture still treats death with taboo, fear, and anxiety. The Analects of Confucius saying "once enlightened, one can die early but happily" conveys that living is to explore the value of life, while death itself is meaningless even be taken as a mean sometimes. A living person must struggle/work hard, but dying means that one can rest, forever.

German philosopher Heidegger explicitly advocated the value of death itself. His "Being-towards-death" brought/showed big wisdom. Living and dying are two separate time dimensions of life and the two sides of the essence of life. When we live, we are practicing life; but we should also know that people are walking towards death once they are born. But in terminal stage, being and death expose to us simultaneously, and this touches us powerfully because "one body and two sides" is illustrated in front of us at this moment. Every day, many people are passing away, and they deliver a message to us, we may authentically become who we are due to our death, but we usually ignore it intentionally or unintentionally.

Modern health care has and unhealthy relationship with death. We are exploring how to make it healthier.

Figure 1   Unhealthy relationship with death.

Available at https://commissiononthevalueofdeath.wordpress.com

Death is a gift from terminally ill patients to our human beings

Death is a gift from terminally ill patients to their caregivers. Each of us has received or will receive this gift. Connecting dying and gifts can help us understand and accept death and prepare for its coming. Mauss's book "The Gift" claimed "the soul of gift", which proposes that people expect the gift but also fear it because they dare not to possess the gift alone. Giving, receiving, and reciprocating are three obligations connected to the gift. It is a mandatory obligation to return with dignity. Refusing a gift implies a fear of reciprocation [4]. There is no way by which the dying person can avoid his death, so Levinas believes that in being-for the other in their dying in the same way that I am with a friend. There is a being-with, a communing, an attending-to, which is an end and value in itself [5].

Our living ones are benefited from the death of others, as well as we receive gifts. However, we cannot return gifts to terminally ill patients because they will soon pass away. We wish to repay, but unfortunately, the other party can no longer receive it, so we express our "regret" in various ways. However, these regrets may haunt us for the rest of our lives. In essence, the idea of the return of a gift to a specific person, is limited, and too narrow. This tradition of return between two individuals is not applicable to the return of the decedents. If we interpret the death of a specific person in an abstract way, we can truly understand that death is the gift of the decedents to our human beings/kind, which suggests a transformation of our concepts about death. If we can change from fear of dying to gratitude for death, then our society can relocate resources of the healthcare and bring more resources for end-of-life care. In this way, everyone can receive proper care in the final stage of life, relieve both physical and mental pain, improve the quality of death, and ultimately promote equality of death. Then each of us will also be a beneficiary.

Reimagining death and dying—the commission's realistic utopia

The report believes that only by recognizing the value of death can we revolutionize the health and death system. In the twelfth part of the report, the Commission on the Value of Death paints a new blueprint for the hospice care and outline its five principles [5]:

(I) The social determinants of death, dying and grieving are tackled.

(II) Dying is understood to be a relational and spiritual process rather than simply a physiological event.

(III) Networks of care lead support for people dying, caring, and grieving.

(IV) Conversations and stories about everyday death, dying, and grief become common.

(V) Death is recognised as having value.

Kerala is a small state in southwest India with a population of 35 million. Of the 2,000 palliative care services in India, 80% are in Kerala. Although limited, at least every district in Kerala can provide services that are estimated to cover more than 70% of those in need [5]. The Kerala model illustrates that achieving such a utopia is realistic. Its success can be summed up in the following: the palliative care services in Kerala were initiated by visionary doctors, supported by civil society organisation, actively involved by groups of volunteers, the long history of social action, the culture of creating a community network of death and chronic diseases, and last but not least, local health policy reformation makes opioids practically accessible.

Table 1   A comparison of whether decedents were accompanied by pain and pain relief in China, UK, and USA

Country	Population (thousand)	Total number of decedents in need of palliative care (thousand)	Consumption of medications for pain relief NME_2011−2013 (kg)	Percent SHS need met by DOME (%)
China	1,383,925	5,501	3,291.6	15.93
UK	64,716	317	7,606.30	523.32
USA	321,774	1,310	167,493.50	3,146.86

SHS, serious health-related suffering; DOME, distributed opioid morphine-equivalent.

Doctors should be the protagonists in bringing death back to life

The example of Kerala has told the world that to change social values on death, a community needs to lead its people to take the first step. Importantly, this change in society has no necessary relationship to the economic development of a society. The report also mentioned the Liverpool Care Pathway (which was an attempt to extend palliative care beyond hospices and specialists into routine care in acute hospitals) in the UK. But it failed to improve the experience of dying. It's not that big hospitals can't provide hospice care services, but the lack of training matters, and should not be financially incentivised. Plus, they must be used as guidance not a checklist, with brains and hearts engaged [5]. In fact, many doctors hold the concept of hospice care, but the medical system and most doctors are often coerced by society and patients' families, and were required to work tirelessly to treat. The subtitle of the report of the Lancet Commission on the Value of Death is "bringing death back into life", and doctors are the helmsman to reverse our relationship with death. For doctors, this is a challenge, but also an opportunity.

References

[1] Illich I. Limits to Medicine: Medical Nemesis, the Expropriation of Health. London: Marion Boyars Publishers; 2013: 190, 205.

[2] Institute for Advanced Study of the Americas. Lancet Commission on Palliative Care and Pain Relief. Background Resources. SHS and DOME by Country. 2018. Available online: https://mia.as.miami.edu/_ assets/pdf/SHS%20and%20 DOME%20by%20 Country_20180410.pdf

[3] Knaul FM, Farmer PE, Krakauer EL, et al. Alleviating the access abyss in palliative care and pain relief-an imperative of universal health coverage: the Lancet Commission Report. Lancet 2018; 391: 1391-454. Erratum in: Lancet 2018; 391: 2212.

[4] Mauss M. The Gifts. Translated by Ji Z. Shanghai: Shanghai People's Publishing House; 2002: 70-4.

[5] Sallnow L, Smith R, Ahmedzai SH, et al. Report of the Lancet Commission on the Value of Death: bringing death back into life. Lancet 2022; 399: 837-84.

主编导读（七）

中国的医患关系：真是无解的难题吗？

中国的医患关系好像一直是一个难题，反复不断地被拿出来讨论和争议。有识之士们提出过许多解决方案，但还是处于一个不尽令人满意的状态。最多就是时好时坏的表象。

我有一个老患者，是肝癌患者，在北京协和医院治疗，经历了手术切除、术后复发、介入消融、靶向免疫等治疗，至今也已经有十余年了，应该是一个成功的个例。老先生也是一位有学识、有教养的前外交官，对于我们的治疗还是非常认可的。半年前，他去加拿大探亲，当地医院接手了后续的治疗。之后从他给我的邮件中得知，他对于加拿大医院医生的关怀、善心和就医环境非常赞赏。虽然主要治疗工作在国内完成，但是我从中体会到对于一个肿瘤患者，医务人员的善意和照顾是如此重要，这种温暖的满足感并不亚于治疗上的成功。

所以医患关系问题并不仅仅是一个医疗问题，同时也是社会问题。它一定程度上体现了整个社会文明发展的程度。只有社会文明和进步有了真正意义上的提高，才能够为改善医患关系打下基础。

具体到医院来说，我们面临的是患者，医患关系可能应该从良好、充分的交流做起。从患者角度上看，他们的确处于弱势，战战兢兢、小心翼翼地来咨询问题，心里充满担心和对于手术的恐惧，但是有时候却找不到主治医生，或者得到几句敷衍的答复，缺少良好的解释和告知。

如果医疗过程一切顺利，那就这么过去了。但是如果出现什么差错或者并发症，加之解释不清或者不解释，就有可能点燃患者和家属的怒火，很多不应该发生的纠纷就这样发生了。实际上哪怕从照顾患者的心理状态、善待患者的职业操守出发，也应该有良好的医患交流和告知。

从医生角度看，也有很大的怨言。工作太忙、杂事太多，除了临床工作以外，又有晋升的压力，还要准备文章和基金申请等；有很多情况下患者确实太啰唆，加上文化教育层次差距的问题等，难以进行良好的沟通交流。实际上社会上各种品行的人都有，好人坏人都会得病，都会来就医。确实有些心存歹念的患者和家属可能给医务人员留下非常不好的印象，有一朝被蛇咬的感受。

我们的社会终将朝前发展，变成一个更加温暖、民众受教育良好、更加理性的发达社会。在这个渐进过程中，我们也得从自己做起，搞好医患关系，逐渐解决问题。

最后讲一个故事，曾经陪同卫生部领导接待美国中华医学基金会（简称CMB）董事长Mary一行，交谈中Mary说她很喜欢中国，所以她居然在家里订阅英文版的《中国日报》，了解有关中国的消息（这在中国人中也很少见）。她想问中国医疗官员一个她不解的问题：报纸上常常毫不留情地揭发中国医疗界一些丑闻，对于医务人员有严厉的批评和痛斥。她说在美国是不会这么做的，主流社会和新闻媒体非常明确，三个社会基本群体是不能从总体方向"打倒""抹黑"的，一个是警察法律队伍，一个是教师队伍，再有一个就是医务人员。她的说法是，在美国也有很多不良警察、医生的做法令人发指，但是从来以个例处理，不煽动社会对这个职业的仇恨，因为整个社会对于这几个基本盘的信任感实在太重要，哪怕是掩饰也比毁掉要好。她原话是我们根本不能担负起这些社会基本阶层信任感的倒塌，社会将为之付出巨大的代价。希望我们的新闻工作者也应该多一些担当和智慧。

本次，我请我们北京协和医院的杜顺达教授写了这篇医患交流的文章，我觉得其中一些观点一定会引来很多反响、争论，甚至批评，主要目的还是让我们重视这个问题，并且努力改善医患关系。

重建中国医患关系迫在眉睫

王禹歆　　杜顺达

中国医学科学院北京协和医院　肝脏外科

在中国，医患关系一直处于紧张的状态且曾呈现愈演愈烈的趋势。仅2009－2018年，中国媒体上报道的严重恶性暴力伤医事件就有295起，有362名医生受伤，24名医生牺牲。

"中国医师协会"2018年的《中国医师执业状况白皮书》显示，62%的医生在执业过程中经历过不同程度的医疗纠纷，66%的医生经历过不同程度的医患冲突，其中以语言暴力为主（约占51%）。

医生对自身职业的满意度明显低于社会调查群体的平均水平，45%的医生不希望他们的子女将来从事医疗行业，侧面反映出医生对目前的薪酬、执业安全、社会认可程度的综合评价较低。

2019年12月24日，北京民航总医院急诊科医生被患者家属以极其残忍的方式杀害，似乎使医患关系到达了冰点。

2019年底新型冠状病毒（COVID-19）的暴发貌似成为医患关系转折的契机。2020年伊始，数以百万计的医务工作者义无反顾地奋战在抗击疫情的第一线，守护着全民的健康，全社会都将医生的辛苦付出看在眼里并由衷感谢。

届时关于中国医患关系的研究表明，在COVID-19大流行期间，中国医患关系有些许改善，医患信任度有所提高。

然而，与此同时，暴力伤医等极端事件仍在频频发生。功能性法律搜索平台Alpha（https：//promote.alphalawyer.cn/）的高级搜索结果表明，2020年医疗损害责任纠纷的总数为18 670件，比2019年增加了约3%，与2018年相比增加了近50%。

此外，清华大学社会学系、中国医师协会人文医学委员会在

《2021年医师调查报告》中提示，从医生的角度而言，医患关系和自我职业认可度没有提高。

中国的医生们，需要时被吹捧为"英雄"，舍小家为大家，无私而伟大，随时随刻要做好上一线的准备；不需要时被"视如敝屣"，被猜忌、指责，遭受暴力，当前这种两极分化的灾难性医患关系发人深省，其背后有着错综复杂的原因。

首先，医疗资源的不平等分配，不健全的转诊系统以及过于侧重科研而弱化临床的晋升制度使得医生，尤其是综合三级医院的医生们工作压力过大、强度过高。

医院等级是国人在就医过程中的一个重要参考因素，普遍患者对大型综合医院的信任程度远远超过基层社区医疗中心；再加上在中国未严格实施转诊制度，导致大多数中国患者无论什么疾病，甚至只是普通的感冒，都会选择直接去综合三级医院就诊，致使综合三级医院的医生临床工作量过大。患者的堆砌亦会导致就诊等候时间过长、接诊时间过短等潜在诱发医患矛盾的因素。

此外，在当下的医院晋升体制下，一位优秀医生的标准似乎更多用科研水平来衡量，如发表的文章数目、影响因子、基金项目等，医生们科研相关压力亦极高。在长期高强度的临床和科研工作下，医生必然容易感到心力交瘁，耐心耗竭。

因此，即便中国三级医院的数量只占所有医疗中心的1.5%，却发生着70%以上的医疗纠纷。

其次，医患关系具有自带负面情绪的特点。人们在发现自己或家人可能生病时，本身内心就已经充满了恐惧和不安，又由于医生和患者在医疗信息中的不对等、国人普遍对基本医学常识的掌握程度较低以及潜意识中一些不正确却根深蒂固的医学观念，都会进一步导致我国医患关系的紧张。

医学知识的匮乏和对自身或亲人的过度关心往往会导致人们对医生有着不科学且过高的期望。

现代医学有其局限性，医生亦非神仙。当不能满足患者或家属不切实际的期望时，极易引发不满情绪。其他许多因素，如医保政策、突发公共事件等均有一定的影响。

很多医保政策的初衷是为了避免出现医生"乱开药、开贵药"的乱象，然而实施过程中，部分政策对医生的诊断和处方有相当的限制，医生需要在看病诊疗的同时，小心翼翼"规避风险"，为患者提供便利或在满足患者诊疗需求的前提下尽可能保护自己，这极大地诱发了医生职业倦怠感。

突发公共事件，如2022年底新型冠状病毒感染实施"乙类乙管"的总体政策后，短时间内新冠感染患者数量的大幅度增加，导致医疗资源的急剧短缺和挤兑。

医院有限的床位被用来接收大量严重感染的患者，导致患有其他疾病的患者无法得到及时治疗。例如，等待器官移植的患者就是受到COVID-19疫情严重打击的患者群体之一。移植前和移植后患者交叉的基础身体条件以及器官平衡分配原则和COVID-19的预防成为新的难题。

媒体在中国的医患关系中扮演着至关重要的角色且有着潜移默化的影响。在新媒体时代，流量和热度成为衡量新闻价值的重要指标，而负面医疗类新闻最是博人眼球。

很多媒体甚至为了追求流量会报道一些片面性的、失实的新闻，并加上惹人关注的标题，类似"产妇死在手术台，医生护士全失踪！""震惊!年轻男性入院2天后死亡!"。但当我们通读整篇报道后，会发现全文并没有对患者的疾病和治疗过程的详细且客观科学的描述。

相反，媒体经常把更多的篇幅放在了患者生活的艰辛或者看病过程的不易上面。这种蛊惑人心却又失实的报道对医患关系的伤害是巨大的。在当今的信息化时代，4小时就足以让负面新闻及其负面影响快速发酵，新闻发出后72小时关注度较高，此后便呈现指数式下降。然而，大部分医生个人并没有实时舆论监测能力，医院大多数情况下会在核实情况后发声，一般均超过72小时。而这段信息空白期，足以诞生各种谣言、猜忌，使消极影响进一步发酵。

这意味着，即使后续对于失实的负面医患新闻有澄清报道，之前失实的报道所带来的负面影响仍然存在，无法全部消除。

当前，很多媒体为了追求时效性不断压缩新闻周期，致使新闻的真实性和全面性无法得到有效保障，近期很多的新闻事实再披露以及不断反转再反转的真相也屡见不鲜。

此外，长期大量误导性的媒体报道让患者习惯性把医生放在敌对方而不是合作方，认为大部分的医生会通过开具一些不必要的检查和治疗来获取更多的利润，并抵制医生所有的检查和医疗建议。

然而，进一步的筛查和检查是协助准确诊断的必要环节。对于这些患者，医生无论有多么高超的沟通技巧都没有办法建立一个良好的医患关系，尤其是在不到15分钟的门诊时间内。可惜的是，这些患者的数量并不少。

此外，自媒体时代的监管不力也是对医患关系的打击。一些有影响力的公众号、微博号以及网站的科普成为当下人们获取医疗信息的主流方式，流传着"看病上百度，买药上淘宝，手术上优酷，边学边手术"的段子。

但是，目前公众号、所谓的微博大V素质良莠不齐，现实中便利店的打印员也可以成为网络上"病毒学的专家"。

大多数网站也均为非专业医学网站，其所提供的信息不准确甚至不正确，抑或与患者的实际情况不完全吻合，每个患者的具体情况都需要进一步筛选和鉴别。

当患者发现医生的诊断与他们从网上"自学"的不一样时，会对医生产生怀疑和不信任，甚至阻碍医生正常医疗工作。

繁重的医疗文书工作一直是医生工作量大、压力大的主要原因之一，这或多或少对医患关系有一定的影响，电子病历系统的发展和广泛使用使医生的日常工作流程发生了翻天覆地的变化，因此电子病历系统对医患关系的影响值得单独讨论。

不可否认，电子病历系统给目前的医患关系带来了巨大的挑战，但是它的影响是正面还是负面的有着巨大争议。

大量的研究表明，门诊时间与患者的信任度和更好的医患关系呈正相关，而因为医生不得不在电子病历上花费大量时间，无形中冲淡了医生与患者面对面交流的时间。

一项研究的数据提示，与2005年相比，2016年医生花费在门诊与患者面对面交流的时间从55%下降到27%，而花费在电子病历上的时间从15%提高到50%。

这意味着在一个15分钟的门诊中，医生花在电子病历书写上的时间大约是7分钟，而与患者面对面交流的时间只有4分钟。更残酷的是，在现实中，亚洲医生每个患者的平均门诊时间只有10.8分钟，甚至少于15分钟。

门诊时间的不足也改变了诊断的模式。由于没有足够的时间倾听患者的主诉，为患者查体，医生更倾向于依赖实验室和检查结果。这种情况下，非结构性疾病的患者和医生之间非常容易引起矛盾，例如肠易激综合征患者。

尽管这些患者腹痛、腹泻等不适主诉很明显，但实验室和影像学检查结果是阴性的，这使得医生在做出诊断和开处方时不得不非常谨慎。然而，这种谨慎与患者希望快速诊断的愿望相冲突，易引发患者焦虑和疲惫的情绪。

当然，如果使用得当，电子病历系统也有益处。对创伤患者而言，医生通过电子病历系统向他们展示CT或X射线影像，可以促进患者对疾病的理解，提高沟通效率，建立更和睦的医患关系。

一项荟萃分析结果表明，大多数研究（22项中的16项）发现使用电子病历系统对医患关系没有影响，5项提示有积极影响，1项显示有混合影响。

医患关系已在很多研究中被证明在疾病管理中起着至关重要的作用，与症状缓解程度和更好的临床预后相关，特别是在需要长期用药和随访的慢性病如高血压，需要综合治疗的复杂疾病如晚期癌症，以及精神类疾病中。

几十年来，医患关系的模式从以疾病为导向、以医生为中心的不对称模式转变为以患者为中心的模式，更加注重了患者的个人意愿。

在以患者为中心的医患模式中，提倡共同决策，鼓励患者在了解不同选择方案以及利弊后参与自己的医疗决策。大量的研究已经证明，共同决策在西方国家有助于建立良好的医患关系，提高患者的依从性和满意度，改善临床结果并降低医疗风险。

而中国的医患关系是相对独特的，相比于被当作个体来对待，患者更倾向于被当作一个家庭来对待，并形成了医生—家庭—患者的沟通模式，即家庭成员共同参与决策。

健康所系，性命相托，面对疾病时，医生与患者是命运共同体，医生勇敢地站在患者与"死神"之间，与患者共担风险，守护生命。因此，医患互相信任、和谐的关系是治疗的重要前提。

鉴于此，中国医患关系的现状亟待改善，如何在中国重建医患关系是一个具有挑战性的社会问题。从医疗体制和医院管理角度而言，医生们存在"自我价值冲突"。

医生是一个职业，但是相比于其他职业，的确更是一个崇高而伟大、有个人价值的职业。治愈患者，守护生命是很直接的价值体现，也是很多人选择成为医生的初衷。

但是在当下的医院管理体制下，一个好医生的衡量标准似乎与临床水平并不直接相关。

而且，大部分医生的薪资和工作强度并不匹配。因此，医疗体制的改革和医院管理的优化是根本。

此外，媒体在医患关系中应该尽量起到监督、推动发展的作用，而非制造矛盾、扩大不满。在如今的社会舆情影响下，医生似乎不能当一个普通人，不是成为被人歌颂的"英雄"，就是成为令人唾弃的"逃兵"。

大面积新冠病毒感染期间，媒体大肆渲染报道医生们带病上班的新闻，成为无形中的道德枷锁，似乎这个时候请病假、没有带病坚持上班就成为一件"可耻"的事情。

医生们卸下职业的光环也都是普通人，也会生病，也有自己的家庭，也需要赚钱生活。很多医生应该面临过这样的场景：照顾陌生患者的同时却无法兼顾自己生病的父母或孩子，对家人的亏欠和内心的愧疚会日复一日地折磨着作为儿女或者父母的自己。

对于医学相关新闻的报道，可以请医学专业人员提前审稿，避免基础性错误。媒体在公共平台上宣传、科普基本的医学知识，有利于提高全民的整体医学素养，也有利于构建和谐的医患共同体。就医生本身而言，医生需要不断提升专业素养，更新知识，了解新研发药物，掌握最新技术。

对于肿瘤和其他复杂的疾病而言，组建多学科团队（MDT），让不同学科的医生各自发挥所长，更有希望为患者提出更佳的治疗方案。

有意提高患者在医疗过程中的参与度，注意肢体语言和沟通技巧的运用，也对建立和谐的医患关系有积极的帮助。

在新时代电子病历广泛应用的前提下，做到完善电子病历的同时，增加与患者的互动，最大限度发挥电子系统的优势，也是新时代对医生提出的更高要求。

此外，在中国独特的医生-家庭-患者关系中，如果能发动基层社区工作者积极参与，可能会对医患关系有所帮助。

基层社区工作者事先收集并完善患者的家庭结构、家庭组成和社会背景等信息，并提供给医生，这可能对医生制定正确的治疗方案有很大帮助，并在一定程度上有助于提高患者的依从性。

重建中国的医患关系迫在眉睫。然而目前的医患关系困境并不是靠一人或者一个群体的努力可以解决的，而是需要整个社会团结起来，从医疗体系、医疗政策、媒体、患者等多方面共同努力，净化从医环境，才能走出当前医患关系困境，重建一个新型和谐友好的医患关系。

参考文献

[1] Si Y. When to end the continuing violence against physicians in China. J Public Health (Oxf) 2021; 43: e129-30.

[2] The Lancet. Protecting Chinese doctors. Lancet 2020; 395: 90.

［3］Zhou Y, Chen S, Liao Y, et al. General Perception of Doctor-Patient Relationship From Patients During the COVID-19 Pandemic in China: A Cross-Sectional Study. Front Public Health 2021; 9: 646486.

［4］Elmore N, Burt J, Abel G, et al. Investigating the relationship between consultation length and patient experience: a cross-sectional study in primary care. Br J Gen Pract 2016; 66: e896-903.

［5］Gottschalk A, Flocke SA. Time spent in face-to-face patient care and work outside the examination room. Ann Fam Med 2005; 3: 488-93.

［6］Sinsky C, Colligan L, Li L, et al. Allocation of Physician Time in Ambulatory Practice: A Time and Motion Study in 4 Specialties. Ann Intern Med 2016; 165: 753-60.

［7］Furness ND, Bradford OJ, Paterson MP. Tablets in trauma: using mobile computing platforms to improve patient understanding and experience. Orthopedics 2013; 36: 205-8.

［8］Safran DG, Taira DA, Rogers WH, et al. Linking primary care performance to outcomes of care. J Fam Pract 1998; 47: 213-20.

［9］Pun JKH, Chan EA, Wang S, et al. Health professional-patient communication practices in East Asia: An integrative review of an emerging field of research and practice in Hong Kong, South Korea, Japan, Taiwan, and Mainland China. Patient Educ Couns 2018; 101: 1193-206.

［10］Stiggelbout AM, Pieterse AH, De Haes JC. Shared decision making: Concepts, evidence, and practice. Patient Educ Couns 2015; 98: 1172-9.

Time to rebuild the doctor-patient relationship in China

Wang Yuxin, Du Shunda

Department of Liver Surgery, Peking Union Medical College Hospital, Peking Union Medical College & Chinese Academy of Medical Sciences, Beijing, China

Keywords: Doctor-patient relationship (DPR); China; media; electronic medical record

In China, the doctor-patient relationship (DPR) has been tense in recent years and continues to deteriorate. From 2009 to 2018, 295 severe medical violence events were reported on social media, in which 362 doctors were injured and 24 lost their lives [1]. According to a survey conducted in 2018 by the national Chinese Medical Doctor Association (CMDA), 62% of doctors had experienced varying degrees of medical disputes and 66% had experienced varying degrees of doctor-patient conflict, dominated by verbal violence (accounting for 51% of cases). Doctors' satisfaction with their profession was significantly lower compared with that among the average social reference group, and 45% of doctors didn't want their children to work in the medical profession, reflecting a lack of confidence in their profession. The DPR in China appeared to hit the bottom when an emergency physician, Wen Yang, was stabbed by a patient's son in an extremely cruel way on 24th Dec 2019 [2].

The outbreak of coronavirus disease 2019 (COVID-19) seemed to be a turning point for the DPR in China. From the beginning of 2020, millions of doctors worked on the front line of the pandemic, and the majority of the public were extremely grateful. A few studies demonstrated that the DPR in China improved and the level of doctor-patient trust increased during COVID-19 [3]. However, this notion has since been questioned. Violence has continued to occur, and the data isn't consistent with the notion. According to the results of an advanced search of Alpha (https:// promote.alphalawyer.cn/), a powerful functional legal search platform in China, the total number of medical damage liability disputes in 2020 was 18,670, revealing an increase of approximately 3% compared with that in 2019, and an increase of approximately 50% compared with that in 2018. Additionally, a survey conducted in 2021 by the Tsinghua University department of sociology Humanistic Medicine Committee of CMDA showed that there was no improvement in DPR or self-professional recognition from doctors' perspectives.

Doctors in China are often praised as heroes when needed while treated with suspicion and subjected to violence when not needed. The current polarization of the DPR in China warrants serious consideration and may involve multiple factors. From doctors' point of view, doctors are exhausted and overly stressed in China, especially those in tertiary hospitals, which lays hazards to the DPR. Because of the unequal distribution of medical resources, the hierarchy of the hospital system is an important consideration for Chinese patients, who trust tertiary hospitals far more than primary medical centers. Since the underdeveloped referral system, most patients choose to go directly to tertiary hospitals regardless of the severity or type of disease, leading to an excessive clinical workload for doctors in tertiary hospitals. The accumulation of patients also leads to long waiting time and short reception time, which are potential triggers for doctor-patient conflict. As a result, it is not surprising that over 70% of recorded patient-doctor disputes occurred at tertiary hospitals, despite tertiary hospitals accounting for only 1.5% of all medical centers in

China (1). Moreover, the current promotion system excessively focuses on scientific research (e.g., the number of published articles, impact factor, foundation projects, etc.) and insufficiently focuses on clinical work. The pressure to maintain scientific output in addition to heavy clinical work is extremely high. From the patients' point of view, DPR carries its own negativity. People are often already experiencing fear and anxiety when they find out that they or their family members may be sick. Deficient medical knowledge and excessive concern for loved ones often lead patients to have unscientific and overly high expectations. Modern medicine has limitations and doctors are not omnipotent. When doctors fail to meet unrealistically high expectations, dissatisfaction may be triggered.

Negative medical news is always engaging and has disastrous effects on the DPR in China. Many media outlets report one-sided and inaccurate news with attention-grabbing headlines (e.g., "A pregnant woman died in the operating room and doctors and nurses missing!"). However, the full texts of these articles often contain no objective scientific description of the patient's disease or the treatment process, instead providing descriptions of the patient's life struggles and difficulties. The impact of negative news can spread within several hours, with a higher level of attention 72 hours after the news is issued and an exponential decline thereafter in the current information age, which means that even if a subsequent clarification regarding inaccurate negative doctor-patient news is reported, the negative impact of the inaccurate report still exists and cannot be completely eliminated. Many media outlets continue to compress the news cycle in pursuit of timeliness nowadays, degrading the accuracy and comprehensiveness of the news, so that re-disclosure of reported facts and reversals of the truth have become commonplace. This style of reporting causes substantial harm to the DPR. In addition, misguided media reports have led some patients to hold the belief that doctors conspire to provide unnecessary examinations and treatments to earn more money. Such patients habitually treat doctors oppositionally rather than cooperatively, and are typically resistant to prescribed examinations. For these patients, there is no way for doctors to establish a good DPR, especially in less than 15 minutes in the clinic, even if the doctor has perfect communication skills. Unfortunately, the number of patients with these beliefs is not inconsiderable. In addition, the lack of supervision in the "We media" era can also negatively affect the DPR. Due to the ease of access and understanding, influential bloggers and vloggers have become mainstream sources of medical information for non-professionals. However, the quality of information from these sources is mixed, and the printer at the convenience store in reality can even become a "virology expert" on the Internet. When patients find that their doctor's diagnosis is different from what they have "self-taught" from the websites, they may question and distrust the doctor, potentially hindering the doctor's normal medical work.

With the development and widespread use of electronic medical records (EMR), the entire daily workflow for doctors has been changed, which poses controversial impacts to the DPR and warrants specific discussion. An increasing number of studies have demonstrated that consultation length is positively correlated with a higher level of patients' trust and better DPR [4], however, EMR documentation dilutes face-to-face time with patients. A previous study confirmed that face-to-face time between doctors and patients decreased from 55% to 27% and time spent on EMR and desk work increased from 15% to 50% for doctors in 2016 compared with 2005 [5,6]. This means that in a 15-minute outpatient clinic, doctors spend an average of 7 minutes on EMR and only 4 minutes on face-to-face consultation. Thus, some individuals hold the belief that EMR has a negative impact on the DPR. However, there are also benefits of EMR, if used properly. For trauma patients, showing X-rays through EMR was found to promote patients' understanding of their disease and increase communication efficacy [7].

The DPR plays an essential role in disease management and has been reported to correlate with symptom relief and better clinical prognosis [8]. The DPR pattern has changed over the last several decades, shifting from a disease-oriented and asymmetrical doctor-centered pattern to a patient-centered pattern, focusing more on patient autonomy [9]. In the patient-centered DPR, shared decision-making is advocated for, and patients are encouraged to participate in their own medical decisions after understanding the options, benefits, and potential harms [10]. The DPR in China is unique; instead of being treated as individuals, patients prefer to be treated as a family unit and favor a doctor-family-patient communication pattern in which family members co-participate in decision-making.

When faced with disease, doctors and patients constitute a community of fate. Doctors often stand bravely between patients and "death", sharing the risk and guarding their patients' lives. Mutual trust and a harmonious relationship between doctors and patients are important prerequisites for effective treatment. Thus, the status of the DPR in China needs to be improved, and developing approaches for rebuilding the DPR in China represents an important social challenge. First of all, reform of the medical system and optimization of hospital management are imminent. Being a doctor is an occupation, but it is also a noble undertaking with substantial personal value compared with other jobs. Healing patients and protecting lives has direct value, and is also the reason many people choose to become doctors in the first place. However, in the current hospital management system, the measure of a good doctor is not directly related to their clinical performance. Moreover, most doctors' salaries do not match the intensity of their work. Second, the media should take responsibility rather than create conflicts or exacerbate dissatisfaction. Under the influence of current public opinion, it seems impossible for doctors to be treated as ordinary people, either being considered "heroes" to be glorified, or "deserters" to be scorned. During the COVID-19 pandemic, the media reported that some doctors were working with high fevers, which became an invisible moral yoke for all the doctors, as if it was shameful for them to take sick leave or stay home from work with illness. Doctors are ordinary people who also get sick, have families, and need to earn money to live. Many doctors have faced scenarios in which they have to care for unfamiliar patients while being unable to take care of their own sick parents or children, and the guilt to their families can torment them as children or parents themselves. When reporting medical-related news, media outlets could invite medical professionals to review articles in advance of publication to avoid basic errors. The media's public platform for promoting and popularizing basic medical knowledge and improving public medical literacy could be conducive to building harmonious doctor-patient communities. Third, regarding the doctor's perspective, doctors need to continue learning, update their knowledge, learn about new medications, and keep track of the latest techniques in their specialty. Doctors who can quickly and accurately make diagnoses and relieve patients' discomfort will gain patients' trust easily and build good relationships with them. The formation of multidisciplinary teams is also a promising approach, especially for treating tumors and other complicated diseases, requiring doctors from different disciplines to use their expertise to jointly discuss cases and ultimately propose the best treatment plan for patients. Intentionally increasing patient involvement in the medical process, paying attention to body language, and participating in communication courses can also positively contribute to building a good DPR. Maximizing technology-related advantages, practicing skills in digital communication, and learning how to interact with EMR and patients at the same time are also demands placed on doctors in the current era. Despite doctors' efforts, fundamental and comprehensive laws should be implemented to protect health workers as well.

It is an important time to pay attention to DPR in China. The current DPR dilemma cannot be solved by the efforts of a single person or group. A united effort is required by society as a whole, including the medical system, medical policymakers, media, and patients, to improve the medical environment, address the current DPR dilemma, and achieve a more harmonious DPR.

References

[1] Si Y. When to end the continuing violence against physicians in China. J Public Health (Oxf) 2021; 43: e129-30.

[2] The Lancet. Protecting Chinese doctors. Lancet 2020; 395: 90.

[3] Zhou Y, Chen S, Liao Y, et al. General Perception of Doctor-Patient Relationship From Patients During the COVID-19 Pandemic in China: A Cross-Sectional Study. Front Public Health 2021; 9: 646486.

[4] Elmore N, Burt J, Abel G, et al. Investigating the relationship between consultation length and patient experience: a cross-sectional study in primary care. Br J Gen Pract 2016; 66: e896-903.

[5] Gottschalk A, Flocke SA. Time spent in face-to-face patient care and work outside the examination room. Ann Fam Med 2005; 3: 488-93.

[6] Sinsky C, Colligan L, Li L, et al. Allocation of Physician Time in Ambulatory Practice: A Time and Motion Study in 4 Specialties. Ann Intern Med 2016; 165: 753-60.

[7] Furness ND, Bradford OJ, Paterson MP. Tablets in trauma: using mobile computing platforms to improve patient understanding and experience. Orthopedics 2013; 36: 205-8.

[8] Safran DG, Taira DA, Rogers WH, et al. Linking primary care performance to outcomes of care. J Fam Pract 1998; 47: 213-20.

[9] Pun JKH, Chan EA, Wang S, et al. Health professional-patient communication practices in East Asia: An integrative review of an emerging field of research and practice in Hong Kong, South Korea, Japan, Taiwan, and Mainland China. Pa-

tient Educ Couns 2018; 101: 1193-206.

［10］Stiggelbout AM, Pieterse AH, De Haes JC. Shared decision making: Concepts, evidence, and practice. Patient Educ Couns 2015; 98: 1172-9.

守在生命的边缘
医者沉思录

医疗技术
何以选择，
不负患者？

主编导读（八）

腹腔镜技术飞速发展的今天，有很多外科医生沉迷于腔镜技术上的进步，却淡忘了外科医生利用这项技术治疗患者的宗旨。

简单地讲，手术的根本意义是为了延长患者的生命。无论什么手术，只有生命延长了，才是好的治疗手段，而外科新技术的应用，也要符合这个宗旨。患者不是供外科医生仅体现手术技能的受体，而是需要让外科医生最大限度地延长生命的个体。

目前有很多文章，尤其是国内作者的文章，越来越热衷于报道他们能使用腹腔镜切除更有难度、范围更广的病灶，手术技能更加高超。当然外科技术的进步是值得肯定和赞扬的，但是目前我们热衷的方向存在的问题是技术进步到底是否真正为患者带来好处。

来自东方肝胆外科医院的周伟平教授就此作出了详细的阐述：腹腔镜技术，我们有没有真的延长了患者的生命？

腹腔镜技术：
我们有没有真的延长了患者的生命？

袁声贤　　周伟平

海军军医大学附属东方肝胆医院　　上海东方肝胆外科医院肝外三科

自1987年Mouret教授开展第一台腹腔镜胆囊切除术以来，腹腔镜手术历经了几十年的发展，各种新技术和新兴设备为广大外科医生们发挥自己的才能提供了广阔的空间，同时腹腔镜手术的适应证也不断扩大。

例如腹腔镜肝脏切除的适应证不断得到扩大，包括全尾状叶切除术、复发性肝癌切除术甚至联合大血管切除重建的肝切除术，大有腹腔镜肝脏切除术无禁区的态势。

腹腔镜手术真的改善了预后吗？

目前，国内腹腔镜下肝癌切除术、胆囊癌根治术、肝门部胆管癌切除术、胰十二指肠切除术等复杂腹腔镜手术的开展日益普遍，但却没有相应的随机对照研究对开腹手术与腹腔镜手术在治疗肝胆恶性肿瘤的根治彻底性和术后生存率的差别作比较。

近期国内一项荟萃研究表明腹腔镜肝癌切除术的并发症发生率、住院时间均低于开腹手术，但1年、3年、5年生存率均与开腹肝癌切除术相当。另外一项荟萃研究也表明对于肝右后叶肿瘤，腹腔镜手术与开放手术的疗效没有明显的差异。

但是两项荟萃研究的数据均来自回顾性研究，没有更高级别证据的随机对照研究，也让这些结论的真实性大打折扣。

同样是肿瘤外科的范畴，国外陆续报道了开腹与腹腔镜下早期宫颈癌手术的对照研究结果，发现腹腔镜手术组患者的术后生存率明显低于开腹手术组，据此提出应取消宫颈癌作为腹腔镜手术的适应证（图1）。

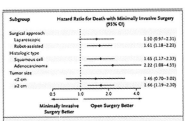

INTERRUPTED TIME-SERIES ANALYSIS
Results of the interrupted time-series analysis are shown in Figure 4. Before the adoption of minimally invasive radical hysterectomy in the United States (i.e., in the 2000-2006 period), a nonsignificant trend toward longer survival over time was noted among women who underwent radical hysterectomy for early-stage cervical cancer (annual percentage change, 0.3%; 95% CI, −0.1 to 0.6). The adoption of minimally invasive surgery was associated with a significant change of trend (P=0.01) and coincided with the beginning of a decline in the 4-year relative survival rate of 0.8% (95% CI, 0.3 to 1.4) per year between 2006 and 2010 in this population.

DISCUSSION

Our findings suggest that minimally invasive surgery was associated with a higher risk of death than open surgery among women who underwent radical hysterectomy for early-stage cervical cancer. This association was apparent regardless of laparoscopic approach (robot-assisted or traditional), tumor size, or histologic type. This finding was consistent across several analytic

图1　开腹与腹腔镜下早期宫颈癌手术对照研究结果

　　这项研究在国内引起了很大的争议，很多国内同行将此结果归因于国外医生手术技术的不足，造成肿瘤扩散或术后并发症增加，而国内医生由于患者人数多，手术经验更加丰富，术后并发症少且肿瘤的根治率更高。但是到目前为止，却没有看到国内医生对自己的经验进行总结，用数据来说服国外同行。

　　临床经验固然重要，但是评价一项技术的优劣不能凭经验，而是靠证据，我们在介绍或者推广一种新技术时应该时刻遵循循证医学的理念，用证据来说话。

"我会做" vs "我为什么要做"

　　国内腹腔镜肝癌切除术年均数千例，涵盖各肝段的切除，但是国内医生大多持有"我会做"的观念，在各种会议上也乐于展示手术入路、出血控制、肝内血管处理等手术技巧，而对手术并发症、术后复发率和生存率与开腹手术有无差别等关键问题缺少总结，还没上升到"我为什么要做"的高度，而后者是更需要以循证医学证据为基础的决策行为。

举个例子，肝脏肿瘤的术后预后及腹腔镜肝脏切除术的难度受肿瘤大小、部位、血管侵犯、肝硬化等因素影响。如何界定腹腔镜手术的适应证？在何种情况下腹腔镜肝切除术后的总体生存率能不劣于或者优于开放手术？上述问题仍应根据不同肿瘤特征分别开展随机对照研究来获取充分的证据，以帮助选择术式。

这就需要通过大量的临床试验进行探索和证实，对于国内肝胆外科医生来说也蕴藏着大量的研究机会。

外科医生们需要怎么做？

外科医生们乐于在技术层面上追求极限，而腹腔镜技术也如期地蓬勃发展；但目前对于恶性肿瘤，腹腔镜治疗技术和治疗原则还没有引起足够的重视和讨论。

相比于切口大小、住院时间长短，评估恶性肿瘤的疗效最重要的指标是术后生存率，只有在保证术后生存率不降低的情况下改进手术方法才是有意义的，而牺牲长期疗效的腔镜技术往往会在后续给患者带来更大的身体和心理创伤。比如临床上腹腔镜肝癌切除术后短期内肝切缘周边出现复发病灶的情况屡有所见，所以对待腹腔镜肝癌切除术的态度需要在循证医学的框架下更加审慎，防止出现技术上的冒进。

我国的临床医生更需要解决的问题是在探索新技术、新方法的基础上及时总结分析，与传统的方法进行比较，发现其缺点进行改进。在此基础上进行证据级别更高的随机对照研究，进而获得更客观可靠的数据，以指导今后的临床工作，为更新或制定新的指南提供依据，这样才能真正使我国的外科水平提高到新的高度。

目前国际上许多指南，如美国国立综合癌症网络（National Comprehensive Cancer Network，NCCN）仍不建议行腹腔胆囊癌根治术等，仅建议采用腹腔镜进行探查。这是因为目前还没有充足的证据支持腹腔镜手术能达到和开腹手术相当的根治性效果。但现状为我们提供了很好的机会，国内的外科医生在这方面有很大的优势，我们病例数量多，能在较短的时间纳入足够数量的研究入组病例，只要我们进行严格的设计和规范的操作，就能在较短时间内拿到循证医学证据，也能在国际上掌握更多的话语权。但是由于我们存在各中心各自为政的问题，如何协调各大外科中心，实现数据公开、资源共享等，进而进行规范化、一致性的高质量的随机对照研究将是外科医生面临的巨大挑战。

参考文献

[1] Vega EA, Nicolaescu DC, Salehi O, et al. Laparoscopic Segment 1 with Partial IVC Resection in Advanced Cirrhosis: How to Do It Safely. Ann Surg Oncol 2020; 27: 1143-44.

[2] Onoe T, Yamaguchi M, Irei T, et al. Feasibility and efficacy of repeat laparoscopic liver resection for recurrent hepatocellular carcinoma. Surg Endosc 2019. [Epub ahead of print].

[3] Wang ZY, Chen QL, Sun LL, et al. Laparoscopic versus open major liver resection for hepatocellular carcinoma: systematic review and meta-analysis of comparative cohort studies. BMC Cancer 2019; 19: 1047.

[4] Zheng H, Huang SG, Qin SM, et al. Comparison of laparoscopic versus open liver resection for lesions located in posterosuperior segments: a meta-analysis of short-term and oncological outcomes. Surg Endosc 2019; 33: 3910-8.

[5] Melamed A, Margul DJ, Chen L, et al. Survival after Minimally Invasive Radical Hysterectomy for Early-Stage Cervical Cancer. N Engl J Med 2018; 379: 1905-14.

[6] Ramirez PT, Frumovitz M, Pareja R, et al. Minimally Invasive versus Abdominal Radical Hysterectomy for Cervical Cancer. N Engl J Med 2018; 379: 1895-904.

Minimally invasive surgery of malignancies: time to argue the fundamental reasons for this emerging technique

Yuan Shengxian, Zhou Weiping

The Third Department of Hepatic Surgery, Naval Military Medical University Affiliated Eastern Hepatobiliary Hospital, Shanghai 200433, China

In recent years with the fast development of new surgical techniques and devices, the indications for laparoscopic as well as robotic surgeries have continued making breakthroughs. In the case of hepatectomies, it could include total caudate lobectomy, hepatectomy for recurrences, and even combined macrovascular resection and remodeling with hepatectomy [1,2]. It appears that laparoscopic hepatectomy has almost no restricted area. On one hand, surgeons are enjoying pushing ceaselessly the technique to the limits, which is promising; while on the other hand, the principle of the surgery for malignancies in this new era has less been focused and discussed thus far. According to the principles of oncological surgery, instead of the incision size or length of hospital stay, the most important indicator for evaluating the success and efficacy of malignant tumor treatment is the postoperative survival time. The King of the treatment for cancers is longer survival of the patients, that has never been or should be changed, and neither to be neglected. The surgical procedure can only be improved without compromising the postoperative survival time. Any minimal invasive technology that sacrificing long-term efficacy tends to bring more physical and psychological damage to patients. In clinical practice, recurrent cancer around liver resection margin shortly after laparoscopic hepatectomy is still seen. Therefore, the attitude towards minimally invasive surgeries requires more cautious under evidence-based medicine, avoiding any aggressive technological movements.

Currently, in many medical centers, complicated laparoscopic and robotic surgeries, including laparoscopic hepatectomy, radical cholecystectomy for gall bladder cancer, peri-hilar cholangiocarcinoma resection and pancreaticoduodenectomy, are increasingly common, but there is still lack of corresponding high quality randomized controlled study to compare the radical cure rate and the postoperative survival of hepatobiliary malignant tumor between conventional and minimally invasive surgery. A recent meta-analysis from China showed that laparoscopic surgery has both a lower complication rate and a shorter time of hospital stay compared to that of open surgery. Also, the 1-, 3-, 5-year survival rates of laparoscopic surgery were relatively equivalent as that of open surgery [3]. Another meta-analysis also showed that for tumors of the right posterior lobe of liver, laparoscopic surgery can achieve the same efficacy as open surgery [4]. It is worth noticing that the data of both meta-analysis studies were from retrospective studies instead of randomized controlled studies with higher-level evidence, which largely reduced the validity of these conclusions. Likewise, in the field of oncological surgery, other authors subsequently reported comparative studies of open surgery versus laparoscopic surgery in early-stage cervical cancer. One study found that laparoscopic surgery was associated with a significantly lower postoperative survival than that of open surgery, thereby proposing indications of canceling laparoscopic surgery of cervical cancer [5,6]. These reports revealed a great controversy. Many clinicians attributed these results to the inadequacy of clinician techniques, which led to the spread of tumors or increased postoperative complications; whereas in

| 守在生命的边缘
医者沉思录

large medical centers, clinicians have more patients, more opportunities to practice and more surgical experiences, so they have fewer complications and a higher chance of a radical cure. In a country like China with a large flow of patients, so far, none of the surgeons has summarized their experiences by using data to convince international peers. Although clinical experience is important, evidence matters more while evaluating the benefit of a technique. While we are introducing or promoting a new technique, we should always keep this in mind: show the proofs.

Nowadays, thousands of laparoscopic hepatectomies are performed in China each year, including any segment of liver resection. However, as a surgeon who performed the first laparoscopic hepatectomy in China, I must say that most surgeons are satisfied by "I can do". They are glad to show surgical techniques like surgical approaches, bleeding control, or intrahepatic vascular dissection, but they lack summaries about the key differences between open and laparoscopic surgery, like complications, postoperative recurrence rate, and more importantly survival rate. Many of the surgeons have not reached the altitude of "why I do it". Compared with the technical level of "I can do", the latter is a decision-making behavior that requires evidence. The prognosis of liver tumors and the difficulties of laparoscopic surgery are affected by tumor size, location, vascular invasion, cirrhosis, and so on. How to define indications of minimally invasive surgery, that is, under what circumstances that laparoscopic or robotic hepatectomy does not have a worse overall survival rate compared to that of conventional surgery, should be performed in randomized controlled studies according to different tumor characteristics. This step requires numerous clinical trials to verify, which contains a lot of opportunities for those hepatobiliary surgeons. Therefore, the problem that Chinese clinicians need to solve is to analyze and summarize in time based on exploring new technologies and methods, to compare with traditional methods and to find their shortcomings and to improve them. Carrying out higher-level evidence-based randomized controlled studies to obtain more objective and reliable data to guide future clinical works, providing foundations for updating or drafting new guidelines, the surgical level can be truly improved. For example, currently, many international guidelines (such as the NCCN Guidelines) still do not recommend performing laparoscopic surgery in radical cholecystectomy for gall bladder cancer. Laparoscopy is only recommended for exploration because there is no evidence supporting that laparoscopic surgery can achieve a radical effect equivalent to that of open surgery. In fact, this provides a good opportunity for us. As long as we design and conduct studies strictly and carefully, we can obtain evidence in a relatively short period of time, thus letting more of our voices be heard in the field. The advantage of surgeons in a country like China is that they have a large number of patients. The studies can include enough quantity of cases in a short period of time. However, the problem is still existed that each surgical center only concerns about their own studies. To coordinate different surgical centers, to achieve data opening and resource sharing, and to perform standardized, uniformly high-quality randomized controlled studies requires coordination on a national or international basis.

References

[1] Vega EA, Nicolaescu DC, Salehi O, et al. Laparoscopic Segment 1 with Partial IVC Resection in Advanced Cirrhosis: How to Do It Safely. Ann Surg Oncol 2020; 27: 1143-44.

[2] Onoe T, Yamaguchi M, Irei T, et al. Feasibility and efficacy of repeat laparoscopic liver resection for recurrent hepatocellular carcinoma. Surg Endosc 2019. [Epub ahead of print].

[3] Wang ZY, Chen QL, Sun LL, et al. Laparoscopic versus open major liver resection for hepatocellular carcinoma: systematic review and meta-analysis of comparative cohort studies. BMC Cancer 2019; 19: 1047.

［4］Zheng H, Huang SG, Qin SM, et al. Comparison of laparoscopic versus open liver resection for lesions located in posterosuperior segments: a meta-analysis of short-term and oncological outcomes. Surg Endosc 2019; 33: 3910-8.

［5］Melamed A, Margul DJ, Chen L, et al. Survival after Minimally Invasive Radical Hysterectomy for Early-Stage Cervical Cancer. N Engl J Med 2018; 379: 1905-14.

［6］Ramirez PT, Frumovitz M, Pareja R, et al. Minimally Invasive versus Abdominal Radical Hysterectomy for Cervical Cancer. N Engl J Med 2018; 379: 1895-904.

主编导读（九）

外科医生学习全新技术时，如何保证患者的安全？

外科领域的技术创新和发展从来没有中断过，而近年来在新兴科技的刺激和推动下，外科技术的创新和进步尤其迅速。临床上诸如腔镜、机器人手术、术中实时成像导航、三维立体成像等技术的应用蓬勃发展；同时一些常规手术、放射、消融等治疗的范围和适应证逐步被扩大到极限。在外科医生们感到欣喜不已的同时，这些新技术在国内雨后春笋般地开展，各级医院出现不加规范和限制的野蛮生长。

一方面这种趋势是正面的，这使得国内的新技术迅速发展，加之病例数量上的优势，使得我国的临床经验很快接近或占据了国际制高点。但是同时，在新技术开展的起始阶段、在准备不充分的医院里，会造成相当高的并发症发生率，甚至死亡率，损害了这部分患者群体的利益。

笔者想说，所有患者的利益都不应该被牺牲。

外科新技术确实应该发展，但是同时如何能够最大限度地保证患者的健康利益免受或少受伤害呢？我们医生的宣言：First do no harm to the patients（首先不损害患者）。这是一个难以圆满的命题。前不久我和安徽医科大学第一附属医院耿小平教授谈起这事，他对于这方面有他的思考和想法。

新技术的发展和推广：
如何在不损害患者利益的前提下完成？

耿小平

安徽医科大学第一附属医院

从1988年首例腹腔镜胆囊切除成功的消息报道至今，腹腔镜设备已发展实现4K超高清、3D和荧光显示。设备技术上的飞速发展，加上医疗设备公司厂家的极力推广，更加促进了临床的快速、广泛的应用。现已经应用到胰十二指肠切除术、各种肝叶切除术和肝门胆管癌联合肝叶切除术等极高难度手术中。同时DaVinci手术机器人的发展和改进，激励了更多外科医生变得热衷于采用这些先进设备去完成各类复杂的手术。

1992年，正是腹腔镜胆囊切除术刚刚兴起的时候，Altman在《纽约时报》发表了 *When Patient's Life Is Price of Learning New Kind of Surgery*，文章提出：当外科医生学习一种全新的手术技术时，如何保证患者的安全？文中指出这种新的外科技术在快速发展过程中给患者带来的意外伤害常被忽视，并被归结于"学习曲线"应付出的代价。强调只有当外科医生对自己传统开放胆囊切除术技术感到自信时，他才能进行腹腔镜胆囊切除术。30多年过去了，现在看来以上论点的细节不一定都正确，但是Altman给予我们的警示仍然是有意义。

但是问题还在：患者的生命不应成为学习新外科技术的代价。我们如何来避免让患者的生命和健康成为新技术发展的代价呢？

开放手术依然有价值

首先要把传统外科手术培训作为新技术推广的基础。

传统外科医生手术培训常经历动物手术、担当手术助手的过程，经反复训练后才能胜任独立手术操作的工作。这有助于外科医生很好地体验、掌握手术相关的解剖特点，了解手术技术难点，掌握手术节奏，在开放术野中亲身感触每一步操作的要点，这是外科教学的精髓。

当我们通过严格的外科培训，充分掌握了手术技术要点后，再采用新的技术，如仅有间接触觉或完全没有触觉的腔镜或机器人设备，才能更有自信地完成手术，也可以减少"学习曲线"给患者带来的伤害。

因此，众多国家的专业学会针对腔镜和机器人外科手术提出了不同的技术准入标准，这些标准主要依据医院的年度专科手术量、主刀医生既往开放手术的数量和质量，经过严格的评估后，合格的中心和医生方可施行腔镜和机器人手术。

实际上，一名具有开放手术经验的外科医生实施腔镜或机器人手术，会比一名没有开放手术经验的医生所经历的"学习曲线"更短，付出的代价也更低。严格的外科培训是开展所有新技术的根本，别无捷径可循。

新技术还是旧方法？合适才是最重要的

要针对不同的疾病或同疾病的不同程度和阶段合理选择新的手术和治疗手段。合理选择一个合适的治疗手段不仅是一个技术问题还是一个社会伦理问题。一方面是高新技术发展和推广的需要，医院、厂家、保险公司出于各种利益的原因也期望开展。另一方面，外科医生也很愿意尝试新技术去完成更具挑战性的复杂手术，在技术上不断完善自己，这也是腔镜与机器人手术快速发展的主要动力之一。

按照常规的心理，外科医生会选择一种自己最熟悉和最安全的手术方法，但是当现在外科医生掌握了三种以上手术技术的时候，即可根据病变的性质、解剖特点和患者的需求择优选择治疗方案。前提是要保证手术安全、患者受益。

目前针对开放性、腔镜以及机器人手术的临床研究多局限于手术安全性和术后近期疗效的比较，对手术后远期疗效的影响知之甚少。

2018年MD Anderson医院在《新英格兰医学杂志》同期发表了两篇有关机器人等腔镜手术对子宫癌远期疗效影响的研究结果。其中一项涉及全球33个医学中心的Ⅲ期研究，纳入了631例患者，结果因发现机器人等腔镜手术后子宫癌的4.5年肿瘤复发率显著高于传统开放手术而被中止研究。

另一项研究是联合哈佛大学、哥伦比亚大学和西北大学分析了美国国家癌症数据库（NCDB）和美国国家癌症中心（NCI）两大癌症数据库的回顾性、流行病学研究。结果显示：接受机器人等腔镜根治子宫切除术后4年死亡风险为9.1%，而接受开放式根治切除术则为5.3%，同时2006—2010年，其间采用腔镜根治切除术后4年生存率每年均下降了0.8%。结论是腔镜手术降低了早期宫颈癌根治切除患者的长期生存率。

这两项研究结果已经影响并改变了MD Anderson医院早期宫颈癌患者的治疗方案和疾病管理。虽然这样的负性结果受多种因素的影响，但这使我们清醒地认识到，腔镜技术可能使患者术后快速康复受益，但远期的治疗效果对患者来说更为重要。因此，对其他专科的腔镜手术远期疗效评估仍在广泛进行中，在得出结论性意见之前应该遵循诊治指南、把握好手术适应证。例如腔镜肝脏切除术，当估计可能已并发肿瘤破裂、门静脉癌栓和可能需要修复主肝静脉下腔静脉时，不应再考虑采用腔镜手术。总之，外科医生在不断追求技术上的突破时更应关注可能对长期疗效产生的影响。

冷静看待，理智选择新技术

如今很多人工智能技术如同在"真空状态"下完成的实验，很难在现实中重现。当我们看到人工智能无人驾驶技术的成功时，便想象不久可能将诞生智能手术机器人，在无人控制下即可独立完成手术。

然而这些理想的高新技术通常是建立在标准状态下的，例如无人驾驶系统运行的前提是有符合规范设置的交通道路和人人都遵守的交通规则。智能手术机器人则需要良好的全景显示和标准的器官与组织解剖结构。这些新技术本身存在的缺陷会限制其广泛运用。

2015年2月英国首例通过机器人进行心脏瓣膜修复术时术中出现故障导致患者术后死亡，在随后的听证会上，主刀医生承认"在一个国家应用这项技术，是一名创新型外科医生希望做的事情"。而他本人却在没有完全掌握机器人性能时操之过急，还没学会走就想跑了。其次，他本应该但并没有告知患者这是首例机器人手术，而采用传统开放手术可能会更安全。

这些都警示我们，高新技术应用的过程中可能会发生的意外在最初设计过程中并未得到很好的控制。高新技术可能会带来新的问题，这些问题必须在应用中发现并加以解决。因此才有了一代又一代的新型设备，使得外科腔镜和手术机器人技术更加完美。但是如果我们回到最初的因高新技术导致意外的问题，如果与传统外科相比，这些新型的昂贵设备和先进技术并不能改善或提高远期的疗效，那还是我们所期望学习和发展的技术吗？

手术方法 vs 远期疗效

目前在不同国家、不同医学中心实施腔镜/机器人手术和传统手术的比例差别很大。一方面与设备条件和经济发展水平相关，另一方面与外科决策医生的认知与兴趣以及手术技术水平相关。以肝胆胰外科为例，普通医院通过腔镜或机器人完成的复杂手术仅占20%左右，但在一些经验丰富的专科中心可能高达70%，甚至更高。

这一现象也许能回答一个较为困难的问题——是患者需要还是外科医生更愿意采用新的方法进行手术？

当外科医生热衷于学习腔镜与机器人手术技术时，要面临"学习曲线"这个不可回避的问题，在复杂肝胆胰手术中这个问题更为突出。例如腔镜Whipple手术最初平均手术时间均＞10小时，且因此导致在一些医院的死亡率较高。不少临床回顾性研究表明，在年度低手术量的医院腔镜 Whipple 手术死亡率明显升高。这也意味着当外科医生学习这项新手术技术时，患者可能要付出生命的代价。而在30年前腹腔镜胆囊切除术初期尝试时，仅仅可能因"学习曲线"就增加了胆管意外损伤的发生率而非手术死亡率。因此我会提议腔镜与机器人复杂手术最好是在严格手术训练专科中心、由经验丰富的主刀医生施行。这符合外科发展规律且以患者获益最大化为目标。

从目前全球外科发展的不平衡状态来看，在经济和技术条件较好的发达国家和地区，可能会产生不少以腔镜、机器人手术为特长的优秀医学中心。

但在众多发展中国家仍然以传统外科为主导，即使在人工智能高速发展的今天，也可以预估这种不平衡外科格局仍将持续很长时间。这也凸显了在高新技术不断发展的今天，坚持发展并改进传统外科技术同样重要，因此将高新技术与传统外科融合发展则可能是一个更好且更为实际的选择。

人类创新是永无止境的，无论你喜欢还是不喜欢，这些技术创新都还会层出不穷的，而我们要做的是如何保持清醒的头脑，不被高科技"绑架"，使我们在追逐学习新技术的同时不断完善外科治疗的长期疗效。

参考文献

［1］Altman LK. THE DOCTOR'S WORLD; When Patient's Life Is Price of Learning New Kind of Surgery［N］. The New York Times 1992-06-23.

［2］Melamed A, Margul DJ, Chen L, et al. Survival after Minimally Invasive Radical Hysterectomy for Early-Stage Cervical Cancer. N Engl J Med 2018; 379: 1905-14.

［3］Ramirez PT, Frumovitz M, Pareja R, et al. Minimally Invasive versus Abdominal Radical Hysterectomy for Cervical Cancer. N Engl J Med 2018; 379: 1895-904.

［4］Droese R. UK's first robot-assisted heart valve surgery results in patient's death. The New York Times, 1992-06-23. RT news, 2018 Dec.

How to balance the development of new surgical techniques and protection of patients' health interests ?

Geng Xiaoping

Hepatobiliary Surgery Department, The First Affiliated Hospital of Anhui
Medical University, Hefei 230022, China

In 1992, when the usage of laparoscopic cholecystectomy began
to rise, Altman [1] published "When Patient's Life Is Price of Learning
New Kind of Surgery" in The New York Times. Altman pointed out
that accidental injuries to patients during the rapid development of new
surgical techniques were often overlooked and attributed to the price of
the "learning curves" attached to these techniques. He emphasized that
surgeons should only carry out laparoscopic cholecystectomy when they
are confident in performing traditional open cholecystectomy. Thirty years
have passed, and Altman's warning still seems valuable.

Since the first successful laparoscopic cholecystectomy in 1988,
the laparoscopic devices have developed to being 4K Ultra HD, 3D, and
fluorescent display under the help from industry. New surgical systems
like the Da Vinci have also attracted more attention from surgeons in
using these new techniques, which have now been applied to many
different kinds of complicated surgeries, like pancreatoduodenectomy,
liver lobectomy, and hilar cholangiocarcinoma resection. The problems,
however, remain. How can we avoid paying the price of harming a
patient's health or life while developing new techniques?

First, we hypothesize that traditional surgical training is the foundation before any new techniques can be promoted. In traditional surgical training, surgeons often first perform animal experiments, then are aided by senior surgeons for more practice on the table before masting surgery independently. This pathway enables surgeons to gain a better understanding of the anatomy, the problematic parts of an operation, and the flow of various strategies in the open surgery field, which is the core of surgical training. Only after this pathway, can surgeons confidently adopt new technologies, such as laparoscopy or robotic surgery, which involve little tactile sensation, while reducing the "learning curve" of harm to the patients. Therefore, in many countries, medical professional societies have proposed different access standards for the performance of laparoscopy and robotic surgery. These standards are based on the annual volume of specialized surgery in the hospital, the quantity and quality of surgeons' past open surgeries. Only the surgeons who meet the standard may perform laparoscopic or robotic surgery. A surgeon with experience in conventional surgery who learns to perform laparoscopic or robotic surgery will have a shorter "learning curve" and thus inflict less harm than those who directly go through training via laparoscopic or robotic surgery. Rigorous surgical training is the foundation of all modern technologies; there are no shortcuts.

Second, surgeons should select new surgeries or treatments for different diseases or distinct stages of the same disease. Selecting a suitable treatment is not only a technical issue but an ethical one. On the one hand, hospitals, industries, and insurance companies expect to develop and to promote high-tech surgeries. On the other hand, surgeons are always willing to try new techniques which challenge their limits. This continuous improvement of their techniques gives surgeons confidence and satisfaction after each success, which is also one of the main driving forces for the rapid development of laparoscopic and robotic surgery. Typically,

守在生命的边缘
医者沉思录

surgeons choose the surgical methods that they are most familiar with, but once a surgeon comprehends more than three surgical techniques, one can choose the best treatment according to the nature of the lesion, the anatomical characteristics, and the needs of the patient. Nowadays, while ensuring the safety and the benefit of patients, clinical research in open, laparoscopic, and robotic surgery is mostly limited to the comparison of surgical safety and short-term efficacy after surgery. Little is known about the long-term outcome after surgery.

In 2018, doctors from MD Anderson Hospital published two studies on the long-term efficacy of minimally invasive surgery, such as robotic surgery, in uterine cancer in The New England Journal of Medicine. One study was a phase III study that included 631 cases involving 33 medical centers around the world. However, it was suspended because it found that the 4.5-year tumor recurrence rate of uterine cancer after minimally invasive surgery was significantly higher than that of traditional open surgery [2]. Another study is a retrospective, epidemiological study of two major cancer databases, the National Cancer Database (NCDB) and the National Cancer Institute (NCI), in collaboration with Harvard University, Columbia University, and Northwestern University [3]. The results showed that at 4 years after surgery, the risk of death was 9.1% for minimally invasive robotic radical hysterectomy and 5.3% for open radical resection. Meanwhile, the 4-year survival rate after minimally invasive radical resection dropped by 0.8% per year from 2006 to 2010. It was concluded that minimally invasive surgery reduced the long-term survival of patients who underwent radical resection of early cervical cancer.

The results of these two studies changed the treatment plan and disease management of patients with early cervical cancer at MD Anderson Hospital. Although the negative results were influenced by multiple factors, it made us realize that laparoscopic technology with rapid recovery after surgery may benefit patients in the short term, but it is the long term that is more important. The long-term efficacy of laparoscopic surgery in other specialties is still being broadly evaluated. Therefore, before any conclusion is reached, surgeons should follow the guidelines with corresponding surgical indications.

Currently, in different countries, the ratio of laparoscopic or robotic surgery to traditional surgery varies between different medical centers. This variation is related to the economic development that affects equipment conditions and is related to the knowledge of medical decision-makers based on the level of their surgical skills. In regular hospitals, taking hepatopancreatobiliary surgery as an example, only 20% of complex surgeries are performed by laparoscopic and robotic surgery, but the percentile might be 70% or even higher in some experienced specialty centers. This phenomenon may answer the core question of whether the patient or the surgeon actually needs new techniques in surgery. When surgeons are keen to learn new technologies, the "learning curve" is unavoidable, especially in complex hepatopancreatobiliary surgeries. For example, in the beginning, the average operation time of the laparoscopic Whipple procedure exceeds 10 hours. Many clinical retrospective studies have shown that the mortality rate of the laparoscopic Whipple procedure in hospitals with low surgery volume is significantly higher, which means that when surgeons are learning this new surgical technique, the price might be patients' lives.

In contrast, 30 years ago, at the beginning of laparoscopic cholecystectomy, the "learning curve" may have only increased accidental bile duct injuries rather than surgical mortality. Therefore, it is suggested that complicated laparoscopic and robotic surgery should be performed by experienced surgeons at specialized surgical training centers. These ideas are consistent with surgical development, and they can maximize the benefits for patients. Based on the current global imbalance in the development of surgical techniques, in developed countries and regions, the number of great medical centers specializing in laparoscopy and robotic surgery will rise. However, in developing countries, traditional surgery will still lead. Even with the rapid development of artificial intelligence, it can be predicted that this imbalance will continue for a long time. Therefore, improving traditional surgical techniques by integrating high tech is essential and might be the optimal solution.

Third, be rational with the development of high-tech surgery. Nowadays, a considerable amount of artificially intelligent high tech is evaluated in a "vacuum" state, so it might be difficult to replicate performances. When we see the success of AI in autonomous vehicles, we start to wonder if AI surgical robots will follow shortly, allowing surgeries to be performed autonomously. However, high-tech devices are often built on standardized ideal conditions. For example, the premise of the autonomous vehicle system is that traffic rules are followed, and roads are in a standard setting. For AI surgical robots, a good full view and an organ with standardized anatomy are needed. The shortcomings of these recent technologies will limit their applications.

In February 2015, a patient in the UK died from the failure of robotic heart valve repair. At the later hearing, the surgeon admitted that "the application of this technology is a thing that any innovative surgeon would do." [4]. However, the surgeon had performed the surgery too soon. Metaphorically, he had wanted to run before he could walk. Also, he should have informed the patient that the surgery was the first robotic surgery he had ever performed and that a traditional open surgery might be safer.

All of this serves as a warning to us for the application of novel technology. Accidents might happen beyond the first design. New techniques may bring unfamiliar problems that must be discovered and addressed during their applications. Therefore, there are new generations of equipment that make laparoscopy and surgical robots better. However, let us go back to the initial question: if the new and expensive equipment and techniques cannot improve the long-term efficacy compared with traditional surgery, are they still the techniques that we expect to learn and develop? The answer is simply: innovation is endless. Whether the public supports it or not, these technological innovations will continue to rise. What we need to do is to keep our minds clear and not being trapped by novel technology, so that we can continuously improve the long-term efficacy of surgical treatment while embracing new techniques.

References

［1］ Altman LK. THE DOCTOR'S WORLD; When Patient's Life Is Price of Learning New Kind of Surgery ［N］. The New York Times 1992-06-23.

［2］ Melamed A, Margul DJ, Chen L, et al. Survival after Minimally Invasive Radical Hysterectomy for Early-Stage Cervical Cancer. N Engl J Med 2018; 379: 1905-14.

［3］ Ramirez PT, Frumovitz M, Pareja R, et al. Minimally Invasive versus Abdominal Radical Hysterectomy for Cervical Cancer. N Engl J Med 2018; 379: 1895-904.

［4］ Droese R. UK's first robot-assisted heart valve surgery results in patient's death. The New York Times, 1992-06-23. RT news, 2018 Dec.

机器人辅助手术，是腔镜手术的必然进化阶段吗？

当今，腔镜手术在临床上已经进入一个非常成熟的阶段，在各个外科领域里以至于在基层医院里，有相当一部分手术是通过腔镜技术来完成的。有些专科适合的手术基本上是由腹腔镜（或者胸腔镜）来完成了，它的优点也非常明确，就是创伤小、恢复快。

回想起来，在普外科最初开展的腔镜技术是胆囊切除术，那个时候有些外科前辈还不是很适应，因为当时强调的是传统意义上的"手术视野的充分展示"，腔镜好似"管中窥豹"，被认为有违外科原则，也不符合当时所谓的"大医生，大视野"的理念。对于这些过程，现在的年轻医生可能已经没有听说了，也感到不理解，因为时代变了。现如今，外科界对于腔镜技术的接受程度已经达到很高的程度，这还是因为它的益处很明确，这也叫实践是检验真理的标准，合理的技术肯定会留下来。老百姓虽然理解不深，但是往往把它简称为"微创"，社会接受度也很高。

而目前，又有机器人辅助手术的技术隆重登场了！实际上一开始设计机器人辅助系统是为远程手术而准备的，即优秀的外科医生可以不在手术台边上，利用操作遥控机械臂来完成手术。这个"不在手术台边上"的优势原来是用于不在同一个医院或者不在同一个城市进行远程手术操作。但是这种原本设计的用途目前没有被真正应用，外科医生基本上是在手术间的外面进行的手术。

原理上机器人辅助手术还是与腔镜手术类同，在腹部打数个孔，通过机械手臂来操作。但是真正体会了以后，会发现它的视野更清晰、操作终端更加细致灵活，机械臂前端部分有手腕的感觉，这项技术慢慢开始受到欢迎。

问题来了，机器人辅助手术的费用和腔镜手术费用没有办法作比较，它高出腔镜手术很多倍（大部分城市目前还不在医保范围内）。那么机器人手术真的是腔镜手术的必然进化阶段吗？也就是它是要逐渐取代腔镜手术吗？它有没有推高整体手术费用的忧虑？

经常有人讨论，机器人手术费用比腔镜费用高出来的那部分是否真正值得花？是否能在治疗的精细和患者的康复上得到很好的回报？目前机器人手术的迅速推广，是不是有一部分来自商业公司的大力助推？但是如果实际上确有好处，那么患者利益也可以和商业利益得到双赢。实际上很多医学的新技术就是在商业公司的推广中变成"常规"的，这种常规同时也给患者带来了好处，那机器人辅助手术是不是属于上述情形的又一个例子呢？

我们知道，任何新技术在开始发展的时候都会受到这样那样的质疑，因为有些颠覆了传统的概念，以至于似乎不可接受。但是随着时间的推移，有部分当年的新技术逐步变成了常规方法；也有一部分技术在临床实践中渐渐式微，最后悄然退出江湖。时间会给出最终的答复。

那么机器人辅助手术技术最后会有什么发展前景呢？是不是会演变成一种可以完全替代腔镜的技术呢？随着用量和例数的增加（或者机器人国产化以后），是不是可以促使单例的价格发生明显的下降？经济社会的发展最后是不是会"稀释"这种昂贵？

就这些问题我们请了国内微创外科大家陈亚进教授专门写了一篇文章，对此进行点评。

肝胆胰机器人技术——腔镜技术的进化还是革命？

曹　君　　陈亚进

中山大学孙逸仙纪念医院　肝胆外科

机器人辅助手术为外科手术展示了全新的视野和流程，尤其在某些特定学科或特定术式上展现出明显优势，继腔镜手术后掀起了新一轮的外科技术浪潮。

回顾百年外科发展的历史，出现过很多次技术浪潮，有的已成为经典和标准，有的仍在不断进化中，有的在实践中被逐渐摈弃。

在腔镜技术日渐成熟、精准，并纳入很多术式的标准手术中的情景下，机器人辅助手术的定位及其发展前景如何？值得政府、医疗机构和外科医生们深度思考。

机器人辅助手术技术是腔镜技术的进化而非革命性改变

经过30年的发展，腔镜技术经历了从探索、质疑、接受、标准化和逐渐普及的过程。随着经验的积累和手术设备的不断更新，很多腔镜手术，尤其是腹腔镜肝胆胰术式逐步实现了可量化、可视化、可控化和标准化的精准外科目标。尤其在有经验的腔镜外科中心，90%的腹部手术可以在腹腔镜下高质量完成。

当然，一些高难度的手术如复杂肝胆胰腔镜手术还存在同质化和普及推广的瓶颈。这主要归咎于腔镜技术的固有局限性，包括触觉缺失、解剖方向迷失、特殊部位暴露困难、止血手段有限、缝合困难以及器械操作角度相对固定和人手震颤影响等因素，导致腔镜术式较开放术式额外增加了手术难度并延长了学习曲线。

此外，腔镜手术中主刀医生的掌控和操作空间更为局限，需要更为成熟和高效的助手团队。设备技术的进步有助于克服部分问题，但并未能完全解决，而机器人辅助技术正是在这样的背景环境下，针对腔镜技术的部分局限提供了改进。

机器人自带的裸眼3D和高倍放大视野可提供更为精细的术野解剖，主刀自控镜头和复合机械臂的设置也在一定程度上降低了助手的技术要求和人力需求。高度自由的器械操作角度和人手震颤过滤，为微小术野的复杂解剖和刁钻缝合操作提供了便利，有助于提高手术完成质量和更快度过缝合学习曲线。

这些优势在一些特定肝胆胰术式上展现得淋漓尽致，如淋巴结清扫、胆肠吻合、胰肠吻合等操作。

更重要的是，机器人技术直接起源于腔镜技术的改良需求，尽管在套管针孔、机械臂等器械布局上需作出一些调整，但是机器人辅助技术在最核心的术式规划入路层面和腔镜技术一脉相承，可以说机器人技术本质上是腔镜技术在科技时代持续进化的结果，其核心理念并未超脱现代腔镜术式的范畴，因此机器人技术能够顺利传承已有腔镜术式的术式规划入路和循证医学证据而得以迅速发展。

但也正因如此，机器人技术目前并未完全摆脱或克服腔镜术式固有局限性的束缚，特别在复杂肝胆胰手术领域并未带来革命性的整体改进。

总之，具有人工智能、组织感知与反馈、自我学习能力的真正意义的外科机器人时代还并未来临，目前的机器人辅助手术系统只是更加灵巧的腔镜操作器械而已，期待未来取得革命性的技术突破。

现阶段机器人技术的合理评价

正如在腔镜手术发展中总是同传统开腹手术作比较，其在良性疾病的手术中取得了更好的微创和加速康复的效果，而在恶性肿瘤的手术中却仍然有争议。尤其是胆道肿瘤的腔镜手术，处理不好很容易导致肿瘤的广泛播散。

目前机器人辅助手术的发展也是在不断扩大手术适应证，几乎涵盖目前已开展的所有腔镜术式，因此也正在开展对比腔镜手术的大规模的多中心随机对照研究。

由于机器人辅助手术开展的时间不长，普及率也不高，目前的研究结论大部分是非劣效的结果，甚至在某些病种的术式中显示出负性的结果，比如宫颈癌手术。最新的微创解剖性肝切除国际专家共识（2021年版）认为在肝切除术方面，机器人辅助手术尚未能获得足够的优势证据。

尽管在有经验的肝胆胰中心某些腔镜术式已相当完美，如腔镜下胰十二指肠切除术，但是在局部操作中，机器人辅助操作具有明显优势，如高难度的胰肠吻合术，胆管及血管的重建等。

同时我们也要注意到目前机器人技术的成本无疑是较为高昂的。先进技术设备带来的成本增加，是医学科技发展过程中必须付出的代价，应科学理性地看待。随着科技的不断进步，设备的本土化和国家耗材集采政策的实施，机器人辅助手术的普及度逐渐提高，使用成本将明显降低；同时，随着经验的积累，机器人辅助手术在整体治疗过程中或将获得时间和费用方面的反哺，在某些特定术式上可以被其带来的明显获益所抵消（如前列腺癌根治术）。

对于大多数一般的术式，增加的医疗成本为患者带来的疗效获益较腔镜手术并未有实质性提升，疗效的成本获益比，才是评价手术技术效果的核心指标。

机器人辅助手术在特定术式中确实有优势，因此需要同腔镜手术搭配使用，而不是谁取代谁的问题。

避免机器人技术的应用偏差

不论何种外科新技术均要遵循规范化、简单化、普及化的发展规律，否则会导致出现选择偏差和医疗公平的问题。

机器人辅助手术是外科技术的又一大进步，但传统开放手术和腔镜手术仍然是目前的主流。

不可否认，很多医疗机构和外科医生都期望加入手术机器人的高端俱乐部，并以此来作为医疗水准提升的标志，有些外科医生也以完成了多少台机器人手术而自豪。

问题是，在一个科室并不是所有的主刀医生同时掌握腔镜和机器人技术的情况下，或者即使是同时掌握这两种技术的医生，都要考虑如何客观地向患者建议最能使他获益的术式，避免以医生个人的擅长来建议患者的手术方式。

商业公司的资本运作因素也不应忽视。科技领域资本的运作并非贬义，科技的发展本身离不开资本的推动。但如果在推广过程中忽视了技术的局限性和适应证，则可能导致损害患者利益的结果，落入本末倒置的陷阱。技术应用的选择，应以患者病情需求为本，以术式需要为本，避免泛用。

综上所述，机器人技术是微创外科技术未来发展的方向之一。

在遵循基本外科学原则和要求的共同前提下，机器人技术与腔镜技术的发展并不矛盾，甚至一脉相承。

腔镜技术易于推广和普及，其累积的术式规划入路方法和循证医学证据将持续为机器人技术的发展提供强大助力。

就目前而言，两者作为腔镜技术的高低搭配，机器人和腔镜技术针对不同的病例和术式需求，拥有差异性的选择指征。坚持以患者利益为中心，坚持基本外科原则和要求，以临床实践主导其进化，以指南证据规范其发展，是机器人外科领域后续发展的当务之急。

参考文献

［1］Huang Z. Minimally Invasive Surgery and Surgery "Evolution". Chin J of Endoscopic Surg (Electronic Edition) 2009; 2: 1-4.

［2］Chen Y, Cao J. From Innovation to Standardization: Progress and Prospect of Laparoscopic Hepatectomy (1990－2020). Chin J of Practical Surg 2020; 40: 158-62.

［3］Chen Y, Cao J. The Impact of Development of Precision Medicine, Evidence-based Medicine and Precision Surgery on Comprehensive Treatment Model of Hepatocellular Carcinoma. Chin J of Dig Surg 2017; 16: 120-3.

［4］Cheek SM, Geller DA. The Learning Curve in Laparoscopic Major Hepatectomy: What Is the Magic Number? JAMA Surg 2016; 151: 929.

［5］Wang M, Li D, Chen R, et al. Laparoscopic versus open pancreatoduodenectomy for pancreatic or periampullary tumours: a multicentre, open-label, randomised controlled trial. Lancet Gastroenterol Hepatol 2021; 6: 438-47.

［6］Ratti F, Cipriani F, Ingallinella S, et al. Robotic Approach for Lymphadenectomy in Biliary Tumours: The Missing Ring Between the Benefits of Laparoscopic and Reproducibility of Open Approach? Ann Surg 2022. [Epub ahead of print]. doi: 10.1097/SLA.0000000000005748.

［7］Shi Y, Jin J, Qiu W, et al. Short-term Outcomes After Robot-Assisted vs Open Pancreaticoduodenectomy After the Learning Curve. JAMA Surg 2020; 155: 389-94.

［8］Shi Y, Wang W, Qiu W, et al. Learning Curve From 450 Cases of Robot-Assisted Pancreaticoduocectomy in a High-Volume Pancreatic Center: Optimization of Operative Procedure and a Retrospective Study. Ann Surg 2021; 274: e1277-83.

［9］Dokmak S, Aussilhou B, Ftériche FS, et al. Robot-assisted Minimally Invasive Distal Pancreatectomy Is Superior to the Laparoscopic Technique. Ann Surg 2016; 263: e48.

［10］Tsung A, Geller DA, Sukato DC, et al. Robotic versus laparoscopic hepatectomy: a matched comparison. Ann Surg 2014; 259: 549-55.

［11］Zhu P, Liao W, Zhang WG, et al. A Prospective Study Using Propensity Score Matching to Compare Long-term Survival Outcomes After Robotic-assisted, Laparoscopic or Open Liver Resection for Patients with BCLC Stage 0-A Hepatocellular Carcinoma. Ann Surg 2022. [Epub ahead of print]. doi: 10.1097/SLA.0000000000005380.

［12］Cao J, Chen Y. Interpretation of "International Expert Consensus on Minimally Invasive Anatomical Hepatectomy (2021 Edition)". Chin J of Practical Surg 2022; 42: 858-62.

［13］Gotohda N, Cherqui D, Geller DA, et al. Expert Consensus Guidelines: How to safely perform minimally invasive anatomic liver resection. J Hepatobiliary Pancreat Sci 2022; 29: 16-32.

［14］de Rooij T, Klompmaker S, Abu Hilal M, et al. Laparoscopic pancreatic surgery for benign and malignant disease. Nat Rev Gastroenterol Hepatol 2016; 13: 227-38.

［15］Kone LB, Bystrom PV, Maker AV. Robotic Surgery for Biliary Tract Cancer. Cancers (Basel) 2022; 14: 1046.

［16］Giulianotti PC, Quadri P, Durgam S, et al. Reconstruction/Repair of Iatrogenic Biliary Injuries: Is the Robot Offering a New Option? Short Clinical Report. Ann Surg 2018; 267: e7-9.

Is HPB robotic-assisted surgery an evolution or a revolution in laparoscopy?

Cao Jun, Chen Yajin

Department of Hepatobiliary Surgery, Sun Yat-sen Memorial Hospital, Sun Yat-sen University, Guangzhou, China

Keywords: Robotic-assisted surgery; laparoscopy; evolution; revolution

Introduction

Robotic-assisted surgery technology demonstrates a new prospect for surgery. Its advantages are particularly prominent in specific surgery divisions or for specific surgical procedures, which has set off a new wave of surgical technology following laparoscopic surgery. Looking back at the history of surgical development over the past century, there have been many technological waves, some of which have become classics and standards, some of which are constantly evolving, and some of which have been gradually abandoned in practice. In the context of the increasingly mature and accurate laparoscopic surgery, which has become a standard operation of many types of surgery, the government, medical institutions and surgeons should carefully consider the role and future development of robotic-assisted surgery.

Robotic-assisted surgery is an evolution rather than a revolutionary change of laparoscopic surgery

During 30 years of development, laparoscopic surgery underwent a process of creation, questioning, acceptance, standardization and popularization [1,2]. With the gathering of experience and the continuous renewal of surgical equipment, many laparoscopic surgeries, especially laparoscopic hepatobiliary and pancreatic surgeries, approach the goal of precise surgery, that is, quantifiable, visible, controllable, and standardization [3]. At experienced laparoscopic surgery centers, 90% of abdominal surgeries can be performed with high quality using laparoscopy. Of course, there are still obstacles in the homogeneity and popularization of some complicated operations such as difficult hepatobiliary and pancreatic laparoscopic surgery. This situation is mainly attributed to the inherent limitations of laparoscopic techniques, including lack of tactile feedback, non-intuitive anatomical operation direction, difficulty in surgical field exposure, difficulty in suturing, limited tools of hemostasis, limited range of movement, and amplification of hand tremors, etc. All of these add additional surgical difficulty in laparoscopic surgery and prolong the learning curve compared with open surgery [4,5]. Additionally, the operating space of the chief surgeon in laparoscopic surgery is further limited, so a well-trained and more efficient team of assistants is necessary. The improvement of surgical equipment may help to overcome some problems, but not all of them. Under these circumstances, the robotic-assisted technique was created to address some limitations of the laparoscopic technique. The robotic instruments have a built-in naked-eye 3D vision system and a high magnification field of view which provide a more detailed anatomical structure of the surgical field. The design of a self-controlled camera view by the chief surgeon and human-like robotic arm movement reduces the requirements

守在生命的边缘
医者沉思录

of assistants to a certain extent. The highly flexible robotic arm design also enlarges operation angles, and the human hand tremor filtering system provides opportunities for operating complicated surgery in a small surgical field, which ultimately improves the quality of surgery and shortens the learning curve. These advantages are clearly demonstrated in particular hepatobiliary and pancreatic surgery procedures, such as lymphadenectomy, bilioenterostomy, pancreatoenterostomy [6-9]. More importantly, the need for robotic surgery directly originates from the shortcoming of laparoscopic technology. Although some instrument layouts such as the Trocar holes and robotic arms, need to be adjusted, the core of robotic-assisted technology, which includes the surgical planning and surgical approach, is inherited from that of laparoscopic surgery. It can be said that robotic surgical technology is essentially the result of the continuous evolution of laparoscopic technology through time. The core concept of robotic surgery is not beyond the scope of current laparoscopic surgery. That is why robotic surgery can successfully inherit the existing laparoscopy surgical planning and continue practicing its evidence-based medicine smoothly [10,11]. However, due to this reason, robotic surgery cannot fully overcome the inherent limitations of laparoscopic surgery, especially in the field of complicated hepatobiliary and pancreatic surgery, and no revolutionary improvement has been made. After all, the time when surgical robots with artificial intelligence, tissue perception and feedback, and self-learning capabilities have yet to come. The current robot-assisted surgery system is just a more dexterous laparoscopic operation device. We look forward to revolutionary technological breakthroughs in the future.

Comments about robotics technology at this stage

Laparoscopic surgery was always compared with traditional open surgery during its development, the former presented better results in minimally invasive procedures and accelerated patient recovery for benign diseases, but it remained controversial in malignant tumor surgery. Especially in laparoscopic surgery for biliary tract tumors, an improper operation can easily lead to tumor widespread. Currently, robotic-assisted surgery is also gradually expanding its surgical indications, covering almost all laparoscopic procedures that have been carried out so far. Therefore, researchers conducted large-scale multi-center randomized controlled studies to compare robotic surgery to laparoscopic surgery. Because robotic-assisted surgery is a relatively new technology with low prevalence, most of the pre-existing studies concluded non-inferior or even negative results of certain surgeries, such as cervical cancer surgery. The latest International Expert Consensus on Minimally Invasive Anatomic Hepatectomy (Expert Consensus Guidelines: How to safely perform minimally invasive anatomic liver resection) believed that robot-assisted surgery has not yet obtained sufficient evidence of its advantages in hepatectomy [12,13]. Although some laparoscopic surgeries such as laparoscopic pancreaticoduodenectomy can be almost perfectly performed by specialized hepatobiliary and pancreatic centers, robotic-assisted surgery has pronounced advantages in small space operations when performing pancreaticojejunostomy bile duct reconstruction and blood vessel reconstruction, etc. [14−16]. Meanwhile, it is undeniable that robotic surgery has a relatively higher cost, which should be taken into reasonable consideration because the paid price also covers the cost of the development of medical science and technological equipment. As science and technology continue to develop, and with the implementation of the national policy of centralized procurement policy for the localization of robotic-assisted devices, robotic-assisted surgery will become more prevalent so the cost of use will be significantly reduced. Over time, robotic surgery may be compensated in terms of time and cost during the overall treatment process. The cost can be offset by its obvious benefits in certain procedures (such as radical prostatectomy). For most regular

守在生命的边缘
医者沉思录

surgical procedures, the additional medical cost of robotic surgery does not substantially improve the efficacy and benefit of patients compared with those of laparoscopic surgery. The cost-benefit ratio is the core indicator for evaluating the effect of different surgical treatment efficacy. As the result, although robot-assisted surgery has advantages in certain surgical procedures, it should be used in conjunction with laparoscopic surgery, rather than one replacing the other.

Avoid deviation in the usage of robotic surgery

All kinds of surgical new technology must follow the general law of development, that is standardization, simplification, and accessibility, otherwise, problems of selection bias and unequal distribution of medical resources will rise. Robotic-assisted surgery is a major advancement in surgical technology, but traditional open surgery and laparoscopic surgery are still the mainstream. It is undeniable that many medical institutions and surgeons expect to join the high-end club of robotic surgery. Some surgeons see this as a sign of improvement in their medical level and are proud of the number of robotic surgeries they have completed. A problem is that when not all surgeons in a department master both laparoscopic and robotic surgery, doctors must consider how to objectively advise the most beneficial surgical methods to patients, avoiding suggestions based on surgeons' own expertise. Influence from business companies should not be ignored either. Business operation in the field of science and technology is not derogatory, and the development of science and technology itself cannot be separated from business promotions. However, if limitations and indications of the medical technology are ignored during the promotion process, it may ultimately harm the interests of patients and enter the trap of putting the cart before the horse. Different technological methods should be chosen on the need of the patient's condition and surgical planning to avoid extensive use.

To sum up, robotic technology is the one of the development directions in future for minimally invasive surgery. Under the general surgical principles and requirements, the development of robotic surgery and laparoscopic surgery is not contradictory. In fact, they come from the same origin. Laparoscopic technology is easy to promote and readily accessible, and its accumulated experiences from surgical planning approaches and evidence-based medical evidence will continue to provide a strong boost to the development of robotic surgery. At this moment, as a combination of minimally invasive technologies, robotic surgery and laparoscopic surgery have different choices for different cases of surgical requirements. Selection based on the patient's need, adhering to general surgical principles, gathering experiences through practice, and regulating practitioners with guidelines are the priorities in the field of robotic surgery.

References

［1］Huang Z. Minimally Invasive Surgery and Surgery "Evolution". Chin J of Endoscopic Surg (Electronic Edition) 2009; 2: 1-4.

［2］Chen Y, Cao J. From Innovation to Standardization: Progress and Prospect of Laparoscopic Hepatectomy (1990－2020). Chin J of Practical Surg 2020; 40: 158-62.

［3］Chen Y, Cao J. The Impact of Development of Precision Medicine, Evidence-based Medicine and Precision Surgery on Comprehensive Treatment Model of Hepatocellular Carcinoma. Chin J of Dig Surg 2017; 16: 120-3.

［4］Cheek SM, Geller DA. The Learning Curve in Laparoscopic Major Hepatectomy: What Is the Magic Number? JAMA Surg 2016; 151: 929.

［5］Wang M, Li D, Chen R, et al. Laparoscopic versus open pancreatoduodenectomy for pancreatic or periampullary tumours: a multicentre, open-label, randomised controlled trial. Lancet Gastroenterol Hepatol 2021; 6: 438-47.

［6］Ratti F, Cipriani F, Ingallinella S, et al. Robotic Approach for Lymphadenectomy in Biliary Tumours: The Missing Ring Between the Benefits of Laparoscopic and

守在生命的边缘
医者沉思录

Reproducibility of Open Approach? Ann Surg 2022. [Epub ahead of print]. doi: 10.1097/SLA.0000000000005748.

[7] Shi Y, Jin J, Qiu W, et al. Short-term Outcomes After Robot-Assisted vs Open Pancreaticoduodenectomy After the Learning Curve. JAMA Surg 2020; 155: 389-94.

[8] Shi Y, Wang W, Qiu W, et al. Learning Curve From 450 Cases of Robot-Assisted Pancreaticoduocectomy in a High-Volume Pancreatic Center: Optimization of Operative Procedure and a Retrospective Study. Ann Surg 2021; 274: e1277-83.

[9] Dokmak S, Aussilhou B, Ftériche FS, et al. Robot-assisted Minimally Invasive Distal Pancreatectomy Is Superior to the Laparoscopic Technique. Ann Surg 2016; 263: e48.

[10] Tsung A, Geller DA, Sukato DC, et al. Robotic versus laparoscopic hepatectomy: a matched comparison. Ann Surg 2014; 259: 549-55.

[11] Zhu P, Liao W, Zhang WG, et al. A Prospective Study Using Propensity Score Matching to Compare Long-term Survival Outcomes After Robotic-assisted, Laparoscopic or Open Liver Resection for Patients with BCLC Stage 0-A Hepatocellular Carcinoma. Ann Surg 2022. [Epub ahead of print]. doi: 10.1097/ SLA.0000000000005380.

[12] Cao J, Chen Y. Interpretation of "International Expert Consensus on Minimally Invasive Anatomical Hepatectomy (2021 Edition)". Chin J of Practical Surg 2022; 42: 858-62.

[13] Gotohda N, Cherqui D, Geller DA, et al. Expert Consensus Guidelines: How to safely perform minimally invasive anatomic liver resection. J Hepatobiliary Pancreat Sci 2022; 29: 16-32.

[14] de Rooij T, Klompmaker S, Abu Hilal M, et al. Laparoscopic pancreatic surgery for benign and malignant disease. Nat Rev Gastroenterol Hepatol 2016; 13: 227-38.

[15] Kone LB, Bystrom PV, Maker AV. Robotic Surgery for Biliary Tract Cancer. Cancers (Basel) 2022; 14: 1046.

[16] Giulianotti PC, Quadri P, Durgam S, et al. Reconstruction/Repair of Iatrogenic Biliary Injuries: Is the Robot Offering a New Option? Short Clinical Report. Ann Surg 2018; 267: e7-9.

杏林 深深
自 沉思

主编导读（十一）

目前，国内临床外科医生存在一种一直得不到解答的困惑，同时对此还有两种截然不同的声音和答案，困惑就是：到底一名所谓的"纯临床外科医生"需不需要做科研、写SCI文章？

一方面，所有的晋升、学位等都需要研究结果和SCI论文，不管哪级医院医生们都不得不想尽办法去做去写。而普通的外科医生尤其是基层医院医生实在缺乏思路、素材或者研究条件来完成一个好的临床科研课题、一篇体面的文章。

在重压下，可能会出现"不得不造假"的现象，有人甚至戏称为"实逼处此"。

而在另一方面，即使是在西方国家，也普遍存在"纯临床医生"的现象，他们就是以看病和手术为主要任务，从来不需要文章也不考虑晋升问题。

到底在中国现有的医疗体制下，需不需要鼓励外科医生去做临床研究呢？

不久前，偶然同香港中文大学的刘允怡院士和东方肝胆医院的沈锋院长谈起此事。两位当时坦言："没有学习精神的外科医生可能不会是一个好的医生。道理简单，你去看全国做科研、发表文章最好的医院，同时一定又是手术做得最好的医院。"例子不胜枚举。

对啊，如果没有科研和学习，知识就会老化，反过来可能影响临床工作；同时，很多外科的创新和发现，是不可能产生于不做学术的外科医生手上的。

但是，在国内目前的外科领域里，还没有达到西方外科界职业构架分工稳定的水平并形成惯例。在这段特殊时期，结合以后的发展方向，外科医生要如何适应？如何做研究？

这个尚未有明确答案的问题，值得我们深入讨论。为此，*Hepatobiliary Surgery and Nutrition* 邀请沈锋教授主笔、刘允怡院士主审撰写出相关的编者按，以此作为引子展开对此问题的讨论。

一名临床外科医生一定要"搞科研",
"发SCI"吗?

杨　田[1]　　刘允怡[1, 2]　　沈　峰[1]

[1]第二军医大学东方肝胆外科医院　肝脏外科
[2]中国香港中文大学医学院

当前,中国的外科医生,尤其是大学教学医院的外科医生,对基础研究普遍较为重视,在很大程度上是因为职称晋升和各类人才奖励,以及对SCI论文和国家自然科学基金等有所要求。

对比大量的外科临床实践和资料,中国外科临床研究的开展尚不普遍,质量也有待提高,主要原因如下。

(1)对临床研究的重要性尚认识不足。

(2)觉得困难较大,例如找不到新的研究方向或突破点。或觉得缺乏条件,例如病例资料较少等而难以付诸行动。

(3)在现有条件下,尚缺乏有效的方法将临床研究做得更好。

针对上述三个原因,我们外科医生应该如何行动呢?

充分认识外科临床研究的重要性

我们应当认识到外科学发展至今,仅有一小部分临床问题得到了解决。外科临床研究的目的是寻找更多、更可靠、更具有普适性的证据,使外科医生更好地了解哪些患者能从手术中获益?使用何种手术方式、在何时使用能使患者最大限度获益等,借此不断改善外科实践,最终造福于患者。以肿瘤外科为例,当前的外科治疗技术已较为成熟,但疗效远不理想。

外科医生如仅满足于施行大型复杂手术,而忽视通过研究去探索这些手术是否带来确切的生存获益,与其他治疗比较的疗效如何,为进一步提高疗效还有哪些措施。那么，其临床工作只能是简单的重复，难以获得最有效的治疗方案，难以实现真正的技术创新和对前辈的超越。

此外，大学教学医院还承担着促进外科学发展的使命。如通过研究证实新的治疗技术疗效更好，就应当积极提供和发表证据，惠及更多同样的患者。

积极创造条件开展外科临床研究

多数中国外科医生面临繁重的日常工作，因此开展临床研究就需要付出更多艰辛。

产生并保持对临床研究的热情，通常是克服困难、创造条件开展研究的关键。当研究成果惠及大众，推动外科进步时，可以催生其更为执着的研究热情，形成良性循环。外科史上许多卓有贡献的外科学家，医疗任务也十分繁重，研究起步也非常艰难，但驱动他们忘我工作的唯一因素是对临床研究的巨大热情。

开展临床研究需要创造的条件较多，其中，最基本的是逐步积累临床病例资料，建立数据库，深度学习和掌握统计学原理，积极参加药品临床试验管理规范（Good Clinical Practice，GCP）培训，以及深度学习既往文献。目前，中国政府对临床研究的资助较少，但并不妨碍多数研究工作的开展。因为研究者可以与同行合作，增加样本量进行回顾性或队列研究；也可以与基础研究人员合作，开展转化医学研究；与企业合作，开展药物临床评价等。总之，思路拓展对中国临床研究的开展至关重要。

开展高质量的外科临床研究

在现有资源条件下，如何将影响研究结果的因素降低到最低限度，将研究结论的可靠性提高到最大限度，是高质量临床研究的前提。以下几点可能有所帮助。

（1）将临床问题视为科学问题

深入细致的临床工作可发现有意义的临床问题，将其视为科学问题加以研究，可能产生创新性成果。但在研究之前必须通过深入的学习、思考和讨论，明确这些问题是否具有实用价值、是否前辈已经良好解决、是否以现有条件尚不能解决。以免进入"一厢情愿"的误区，这也是既往大量失败的临床研究总结出的教训。

（2）挑战或弥补指南或共识的不足

原始性地创新治疗观点或技术固然值得追求，但对前辈的工作进行技术改进也是重要方向。精读和理解相关的指南或共识，从中发现争议性的、不确定的或未知的问题，可能形成创新性研究方向，获得高影响力成果，并促进指南或共识的修订。

（3）批判性地评估前辈发表的文献

精读代表性文献，努力发现这些工作在研究方法、数据利用、对照设定、终点指标和统计分析等方面存在的问题，尤其是检验其研究内容与结论之间的因果关系是否成立，对提升自己的研究质量至关重要。对此，《克氏外科学》（第20版）第8章有较详尽的阐述。

（4）汲取基础和转化医学研究成果

1）目前，基于各种组学的精准医学研究发展迅猛，"分子外科"已逐渐进入外科医生的视野。将基础研究的结果进行临床转化，结合临床病例资料，可以催生更高质量的临床研究。以肿瘤外科治疗为例，传统的分期治疗原则可能随着肿瘤分子分型的出现而被更新，并且已在某些实体肿瘤如胃癌、乳腺癌中得到初步实现。

2）"选择种果树而非种水稻"。前者每年都可收获果实，而后者只要一年不种就不会有收获。高质量的临床研究必须具有良好的基础和长远规划。系统性的，而非随着兴趣而转移方向的研究，对提高科研工作效率，催生高影响力成果至关重要。

3）让国际同行了解自己的工作。多数临床研究的结果以论文的形式展示，因此准确、精练和质朴的写作特点成为决定研究质量以及使中国的研究走向世界的关键要素。外科医生完全可以通过广泛阅读文献、亲力亲为地长期实践，最终发表高水准论文。

裴法祖教授在《做人、做事、做学问》一文中谆谆告诫外科医生，要杜绝科研作风不够严谨的现象。树立严谨的科学作风，对保证研究质量和我国外科学研究的国际声誉具有重大意义。

参考文献

[1] Simianu V, Farjah F, Flum D. Evidence-Based Surgery: Critically Assessing Surgical Literature. In: Townsend C, Beauchamp D, Evers M, et al. Sabiston Textbook of Surgery: the biological basis of modern surgical practice-20th Edition 2016: 173-86.

[2] Zhou WP, Shen F, Cheng SQ, et al. The way of thinking decides exit and the innovation leads future: practice and implementation of Academician Lau Wan Yee's research ideas. Chin J Digest Surg 2018; 17: 51-4.

[3] Qiu FZ. Behavior, Work, and Knowledge. Chin Med Ethics 2008; 1: 3-5.

Creating favorable conditions for increased quantity of high-quality clinical studies in surgery

Yang Tian[1], Lau Wan Yee[1,2], Shen Feng[1]

[1]Department of Hepatic Surgery, The Eastern Hepatobiliary Surgery Hospital, Second Military Medical University (Naval Medical University), Shanghai 200438, China
[2]Faculty of Medicine, The Chinese University of Hong Kong, Hong Kong, SAR, China

Nowadays, surgeons in China, especially those who are working in teaching hospitals affiliated to universities, concentrate their research efforts in basic researches mainly because these researches can generate scientific articles in journals of high impact factors which are essential for career advancement, job promotion and securing research grants. Clinical surgical research is generally considered as less important because the influence of generating evidence on clinical practice has not been fully recognized by clinicians in China. Furthermore, there is a relative lack of financial and administrative support for clinical surgical research. Finally, surgeons in China in general need to further improve the knowledge and means to conduct good clinical research.

This commentary mainly focuses on these issues.

Fully acknowledge the importance of clinical surgical research

Even with rapid advances in surgery in the recent few decades, it is undeniable that only a fraction of clinical problems has been resolved. The purpose of clinical research in surgery is to establish reliable evidences that enable surgeons to apply to improve their surgical practices. Proper update and advice on surgical knowledge and skills would benefit patients, especially those suffering from malignant diseases. Although oncological surgery is currently quite well-developed, there are still a lot of rooms for improvement. If surgeons are satisfied with carrying out routine and repetition surgical procedures day in and day out, there will not be any further advances in surgery. Surgery advances through innovations in ideas and techniques through surgical research.

Teaching hospitals are responsible for generating innovations. Any new treatment idea or technique generated through clinical research should be broadly promoted to other clinicians so that more patients can benefit.

To actively create favorable conditions for clinical surgical research

Most surgeons working in China are currently overloaded by their daily clinical duties. As a consequence, extra efforts have to be paid in conducting clinical research. To develop a passion for clinical research is the key to overcome all the hurdles in research. The biggest reward for a surgeon-scientist is to produce research results which benefit patients. This reward brings more enthusiasm to do more researches, thus forming a virtuous circle. Throughout the history of surgery, most successful surgeon-scientists have been overloaded with work duties, and their initial research paths have not been smooth. Yet, their great passions for clinical research have been driving them through all difficulties to overcome all hurdles.

Well-designed clinical studies have many steps. The first step is to collect clinicopathological data of patients to establish a database. Then, the knowledge in statistics has to be mastered. Surgeons should also actively participate in the training in Good Clinical Practice (GCP) and learn to thoroughly review the medical literature on the topics related to their research interest. Currently, funding for clinical research from the government is relatively insufficient, but it should not stop surgeons from launching their research works. Surgeons can cooperate with colleagues from other centers to increase sample sizes in retrospective or prospective cohort studies, cooperate with basic researchers to conduct translational medical research and coordinate with pharmaceutical enterprises to conduct clinical researches on drugs. To keep an open mind and to be able to gather better financial, human and data resources are crucial in good clinical researches.

Conducting high-quality clinical research in surgery

The prerequisites for a high-quality clinical study are to minimize biases that potentially affect outcomes and to maximize reliability of results of the study. The following points may be important to achieve these aims:

(I) To solve a clinical problem as a scientific problem. Dedication to clinical works helps to resolve meaningful clinical problems in a scientific way. It is important to treat any clinical problem as a scientific problem. Conducting researches to resolve a clinical problem may bring innovative results. Before starting on any research, surgeons must study, consider, discuss thoroughly, and clarify whether the research project has a practical and meaningful value. Ask the following important questions: Whether the problem has been solved in previous studies? Can the problem be solved with the resources and conditions currently available? A lesson which has been learned in many previously failed clinical studies is: do not have any unrealistic "false hope" on research outcomes.

(II) Fill in the gaps in guidelines or consensus. In addition to creating original knowledge or treatment methods as mentioned above, improving previous works by other surgeons is also a good direction. Find controversial or unclear topics by carefully reading published guidelines or consensus. Innovative research directions to achieve impactful results can be obtained by revising established guidelines or consensus.

(Ⅲ) Critically evaluate previous works by other surgeons. Carefully read the representative works by other surgeons. Find out the deficiencies in their study methods, data collection, endpoint indicators or statistical analysis. In particular, test to see whether any causal relationship stands in their research content and conclusion. Young surgeons may find this especially helpful in improving the quality of their research. Chapter 8 of the Sabiston Textbook of Surgery (20th Edition) has a thorough explanation on this point [1].

(Ⅳ) Make use of basic research outcomes to conduct translational clinical researches. Precision medicine has currently developed rapidly based on various "omics", and "molecular surgery". Translating basic into clinical research can generate excellent research articles. A good example is in surgical treatment of cancer. A number of treatments based on the traditional staging systems have now been replaced by new molecular subtyping.

(Ⅴ) Plant fruit trees instead of corps. Fruit trees take years to grow. However, once they mature, fruits can be repeatedly harvested on a yearly basis. On the other hand, corns can only be harvested one time. To produce high-quality clinical researches should follow the way in planting a fruit tree, and then to develop the planted fruit trees into a forest. This requires a good foundation and long-term planning. Instead of frequent shifting research directions, one should conduct researches around some topics in a systematic manner, which is crucial in improving the quality and quantity of researches, thus generating impactful results [2].

(Ⅵ) Let the peers know your research works. Most clinical studies are published in journals. Good research writing is part of the quality of a good research study. Surgeons should widely read scientific articles, learn to write high-quality papers, and publish more research works so that more peers get to know your research works.

In the article "Behavior, Work, and Knowledge", Professor Fazu Qiu suggested surgeons should be very meticulous in doing researches [3]. Establishing rigorous research criteria is important for a surgeon to carry out high-quality researches and to help him/her to establish good reputation in the surgical field.

References

[1] Simianu V, Farjah F, Flum D. Evidence-Based Surgery: Critically Assessing Surgical Literature. In: Townsend C, Beauchamp D, Evers M, et al. Sabiston Textbook of Surgery: the biological basis of modern surgical practice-20th Edition 2016: 173-86.

[2] Zhou WP, Shen F, Cheng SQ, et al. The way of thinking decides exit and the innovation leads future: practice and implementation of Academician Lau Wan Yee's research ideas. Chin J Digest Surg 2018; 17: 51-4.

[3] Qiu FZ. Behavior, Work, and Knowledge. Chin Med Ethics 2008; 1: 3-5.

主编导读（十二）

尽管我们现有的住院医师培训体系拥有其根据国情建立起来的特色，但一直以来是一个不尽完善、争论不休的问题。

包括设置该培训体系的管理者和接受该培训体系的年轻医生们，都因为角度和身份的不同而对其持有一定想法和感到不尽满意。

曾经有一段时间，我国的住院医师培训制度试图大幅度借鉴西方的经验，学习西方实行了多年的体系，但是很快却又发现直接照搬有"水土不服"之忧虑。

我们的医学生从毕业后进入医院做住院医师起，实际上就是这个医院的在职员工了。其原因之一是即便经过住院医师培训发现该年轻医生并非医院所想要的，对于医院来说，"辞退"过程是很困难、复杂的。

同样地，对于年轻医生，他们经过最初实践以后发现该医院不适合自己，或者自己根本就不适合医生职业，转到其他医院或行业就要经历"跳槽"。而当前大部分医院更愿意留下本院、本校毕业生的做法，导致了"生源单调闭塞"的不良后果，限制了国内各大医院的技术、理念、人员的广泛交流。

培训住院医师的成本和投入也是一个问题，前期投入（包括时间和精力的投入）能不能同后期的收入相匹配呢？如何能够稳定年轻医生的队伍，让社会上最为优秀的一批人留在医生队伍里？住院医师是应该在各个科室经历广泛训练（非常耗时）还是应该尽快接受专科训练？

问题太多、太复杂了，不是通过讨论能够解决的。很多问题可能最后只能在社会的总体发展中慢慢消化并得以解决。

但是我们关于这方面的讨论肯定是有益的，希望借此文章引发我国住院医师对与自身息息相关的培训制度的探讨和思考。我邀请了北京协和医院的青年才俊花苏榕医生写下他对我国住院医师培训制度的困惑和思考。《中国外科住院医师培训：向左？向右？还是向前？》一经发表，收到了7400多名来自国内外年轻医生的留言，他们提出了很多意见、建议以及疑惑。花苏榕医生整理了收到的问题和质疑，并结合自己中美两国规培的经验和思考进一步撰写了《中国外科住院医师培训：你说、我说、他说》，为广大读者做了总体答复。

笔者认为，花医生亲身经历了该培训制度的发展同时也切身感受过美国的培训体系。编写本篇的目的，其一是我想让年轻医生发声而不是让管理者"居高临下"地教育；其二是文章所提到的问题可能涵盖不了各层级医院以及不同专业医生们的问题和困惑，所以也欢迎年轻医生们广泛发声，共同为我国的住院医师培训制度献计献策！

中国外科住院医师培训：
向左？向右？还是向前？

花苏榕

北京协和医院　基本外科

管理部门或许觉得住培的执行力度还不够"狠"，而有些年轻的外科医生却在住培中迷茫并考虑转行。怎么破？不妨把住培看作一款由管理部门推出、年轻医生购买、用于治疗患者的手术刀，看看这把"住培刀"是打造得太复杂了？太奢华了？抑或存在别的不足。

医生的培养成本昂贵

正如生命和健康的宝贵性一样，医生的培养成本是昂贵的，外科尤其如此。

教学耗费带教医生大量的本可用于诊疗的时间，且优秀的带教医生往往身价不菲；外科手术指导需要带教医生付出更多的心血、承担额外的风险；各种模拟培训系统更是耗财力。一套好的教学体系必然要对上述成本予以恰当的鼓励和回报，除非带教医生都是圣人。我们且把"如何设计教学激励机制"放在一边，因为激励教学是需要资源的，而且是大量的资源。

此外，医疗中所有的成本最终都由社会承担。医生的学习培训时间越长、要求越高，成本就越高，"住培刀"就会越昂贵，将来终会体现在医疗消费水平中。强行控制医疗消费水平？如果迫使年轻医生花10万元买了一把"住培刀"，但每次使用只能收10元，那么短期结果是消极怠工、医疗质量下降，远期将导致从业人员数量和整体水平下降。医疗问题的本质核心仍是社会经济问题。

国情决定住培形态

拿医疗卫生支出在GDP中的占比来说，美国为17.06%，人均9403美元；我国为5.15%，人均420美元；世界平均水平为9.90%。

美国医学生需要支付高昂的学费，而且国家管理部门支付给医院高额的经费以换取住培医生的培训机会。医院拿钱手软，加之失去住培基地资格还意味着失去大量廉价劳动力，因此美国住培医生可以挺直腰杆争取自己受培训的权益和动手机会。

而我国医疗卫生支出较低，医学教育投入更低，负责打造"住培刀"的基地医院拿不到多少经费，对带教医生既没有有效的约束，也缺乏有效的激励，这样打造出的"住培刀"质量堪忧。住培医生付出了大量的时间和机会成本购买了这把"住培刀"，但由于自身没花钱、未来就业压力大，在医院只能"寄人篱下"、"仰人鼻息"、埋头干活，无法要求受培训的权益，更何谈争取动手机会了。这样毕业后拿着"住培刀"的外科医生，未必就比过去拿着"江湖刀"（自学成才的）、"进修刀"（带着明确目的去大医院或国外进修学习的）的医生有竞争力。

当然，美国9403美元的"住培刀"也面临这样或那样的问题，我国买不起，也不需要照搬美国的"住培刀"。事实上本着学以致用的原则，我国过去的"住培刀""进修刀"用最低的经济成本创造了极大的卫生奇迹，我国患者做个常规手术和美国相比又快又便宜，质量也不差。

那么有物美价廉的"江湖刀"和"进修刀"，我们还是否需要"住培刀"？这就像专科技术教育和本科教育的差别一样，系统而扎实的基本理论、多学科的基础知识、熟练掌握的基本技能，是外科医生未来成长的基石。

然而，也就像本科生毕业找工作的困境一样，"住培刀"的动手实战技能不如别人，其基本功和综合素质的优势（如果有的话）也还需要时间来发酵。"十年树木，百年树人"，住培是一项长期投资，短期是看不到收益的。

何去何从？

向左？照搬美国模式，一如在1949年想在全国瞬间普及本科教育的愿景，但是我国没有那么多带教储备，医生付不起那么高昂的学费，人民也看不起那么高成本培养出来的医生。与当年普及本科的同时举办夜校的模式一样，大多数外科医生会在工作中寻找性价比最高的、适合自己的培训机会，例如有针对性的进修。

想不增加成本和投入就获得良好的教学产出？天下没有免费的午餐。一如为了本科而本科，如果为了住培而住培，会因为缺少优秀的带教医生、基本的资源投入和成熟的教学系统，无法达到住培的效果，反而浪费了年轻医生的黄金学习工作时间。

向右？我国飞速发展的经济和人民日益增长的医疗需求，显然不允许医疗行业原地踏步。改革的步子迈得太大固然不行，太小更不行。加之我国幅员辽阔，地域差异大，如何动态地、个性化地设计适合我国的"住培刀"款式，是考验管理部门的一道难题。

向前看，各专科大发展的时代逐渐过去。在一个普遍人口老龄化的未来，患者同时有多部位、多系统疾病的比例将大大增加。医疗系统从综合性走向专科化，必然将再次走向综合。近年来兴起的多学科综合治疗（MDT）就是明证，而这也正是在住培期间打牢基础的意义所在。

向前想，对患者而言，经济能力的增长意味着渴望更好的"住培刀"；对于年轻医生而言，医疗需求的迅速增加意味着自己将来很可能成为稀缺资源。在如今有限的医疗预算中，整体上用于诊疗多而教学少，这无可厚非。但对个体而言，受培训的机会是可以自己争取甚至创造的，这些知识和技能就是未来的稀缺资源。

向前走吧，你对手里的"住培刀"是否满意？

参考文献

［1］World Health Organization Global Health Expenditure database. Current health expenditure (% of GDP). Available online: https://data.worldbank.org.cn/indicator/SH.XPD.CHEX.GD.ZS

Residency training in China versus the USA: puzzling the way ahead

Hua Surong

Department of General Surgery, Peking Union Medical College Hospital, Chinese Academy of Medical Sciences, Beijing, China

While Chinese medical management departments may feel that the residency training program is not sufficiently rigorous, some young surgeons may find their residency in the hell mode and consider career changes. What can account for this contradiction?

As much as life and health are precious, so is residency training expensive, especially for surgical residents. Prestigious surgical educators are often paid high wages because teaching consumes much of their time that would otherwise be used for patients. Practical guidance during surgery generally requires more effort and entails extra risk for surgical teachers. Additionally, a considerable amount of funding is spent on various simulation training systems. China is still in an exploratory stage of a well-functioning system that can provide appropriate incentives and rewards for surgical educators. Determining how to design a teaching incentive system is beyond the scope of our discussion. An incentive system requires an enormous amount of financial support, and medical costs must ultimately be borne by society through taxation. The medical system will require more funding as a higher standard for surgeons, and thus a longer training period, are demanded from residency programs. This increasing cost will eventually be reflected in the future medical expense of the patients. However, controlling medical system funding by reducing residents' wages is not viable, as it will lead to both a decline in healthcare quality and in the quantity of practitioners.

China's national conditions determine the level of our residency training programs. The health expenditure in the United States accounts for 17.06% of their GDP, with a per capita of 9,403 US dollars, while that of China is 5.15%, with a per capita of 420 US dollars; the world average is 9.90% [1]. Medical students in the United States pay high tuition fees. The Accreditation Council for Graduate Medical Education (ACGME) funds residency positions throughout the country. In the United States, teaching hospitals or tertiary medical centers not only benefit from having residency programs but also gain financially from having a pool of cheap labor; losing qualification thus means losing both of these benefits. Therefore, residents in the USA can directly request proper training and hands-on practice, as these are their rights. However, China's health expenditures are low, and the portion allotted to medical education is even lower. In contrast to their American counterparts, teaching hospitals in Chinese residency training programs cannot receive sufficient funding. Without adequate resources, teaching surgeons lack motivation and incentive, which leads to the lower educational quality of their residency programs. Although Chinese residents pay a substantial amount of time and opportunity cost to participate in programs, they face future employment and social pressure. They are also hesitant to speak up for themselves to fight for more training opportunities, and many of them are recruited by the teaching hospital to do redundant or menial work. Lacking sufficient experience in the operating room or wards, young surgeons who graduate from these residency programs may be less competent in terms of surgical skills compared with other visiting surgeons (from tertiary hospitals or overseas) or past self-taught surgeons.

In addition to the above, China found it challenging when trying to copy the $9,403 US residency program because it cannot afford the cost of such a program. In the past, it was shown that the low-cost mode of self-taught surgeons and visiting surgeons worked well in the Chinese healthcare system. A routine operation at the same level of efficacy is even faster and cheaper to access in China than in the United States. Does having low-cost, self-taught surgeons and visiting surgeons render residency programs unnecessary? When a career and technical education (CTE) can prepare students for specialized jobs in a short period of time, is undergraduate education still worthwhile? The answer seems obvious. However, an excellent surgeon does not only require the necessary surgical skills but must also possess a broad range of multidisciplinary medical knowledge, which can lay the foundation for future career development. A residency program is needed, therefore, but in a different form.

Should we consider reforming our residency program according to the US standard? If we adopt the US residency program, residents could not afford and would not be willing to pay for such high tuition fees, and the patients could not afford surgeons raised that way. Most Chinese surgeons would look for the most cost-effective and suitable training program elsewhere. Meanwhile, if the US residency program were copied minus the high-quality teaching team and the mature teach-learn system, the program would not achieve the same results as that of the US program, and would waste the time and learning opportunities of our future surgeons.

The question remains then as to what degree reform should be enacted. The medical industry in China is expanding in pace with the growth of economy and the population's medical needs, and residency programs must also keep in stride with this progress. China has a large population base and large geographical differences, and so reforms should neither be too radical nor too conservative. How to customize a residency program that is suitable for China is an indeed challenging problem.

The model of independent development of different departments within the hospital has become outmoded. In a future with an aging society, the proportion of patients with multiple system diseases will be much higher. From an all-inclusive to a specialized model, the medical system will inevitably be integrated again. The rise of multiple disciplinary teams (MDTs) in recent years is clear proof that young surgeons should lay a solid foundation during their residency training.

The rise in social wealth has led to a greater patient demand for a better medical experience. For young doctors, this rapid increase in medical demand means that high-quality doctors will be more needed in the future. In the currently limited medical budget, more funds are used for diagnosis and treatment than for teaching. Thus, for individual doctors, learning opportunities need to be acquired or created by their own enterprise.

What do you think of your residency program?

References

[1] World Health Organization Global Health Expenditure database. Current health expenditure (% of GDP). Available online: https://data.worldbank.org.cn/indicator/SH.XPD.CHEX.GD.ZS

中国外科住院医师培训：你说、我说、他说

花苏榕

北京协和医院　基本外科

《中国外科住院医师培训：向左？向右？还是向前？》发表后，许多不同地区、不同层级医院的规培中或已完成规培的读者来信，总体来说有以下几种声音和看法。

缺乏螺旋式上升的通道

中美的住培体系差异谈起来总是让人津津乐道，无论从纸面的制度上，还是具体的落实上可讨论的太多。从效果上说，中国R1（住院医师1年）和美国R1的起点差距并不大，仅从动手能力方面来说，都是刚刚会缝皮、打结，写病历、换药、拉钩。但是在美国，R3（住院医师3年）就开始主刀做阑尾和胆囊相关手术，R5（住院医师5年）已经能主刀做大手术，甚至胰十二指肠切除术了；而在中国，R3、R5大都仍然在写病历、换药、拉钩，主刀做过小手术的人寥寥无几，更遑论大手术了。

这种差异显然不能仅用"美国学医的人更聪明勤奋"或者"美国聪明勤奋的人都去学医了"来解释。中国住院医师长年原地踏步、重复劳动消磨了年轻人的锐意进取心，蹉跎了学习和练手的黄金年龄，是住院医师抱怨最多的"槽点"，也是许多青年才俊选择离开医生岗位的原因之一。

笔者认为，对于教学管理者，把一个大目标分解成若干中目标，再分解成许多小目标，并且给每个小目标设立明确的评价指标和达成后的奖励，这种方法也许从心理学上有助于学员循序渐进地"闯关升级"。

关于螺旋式上升的教学，从课程体系设计、执行，到反馈和改良均有相关文献报道，在此不赘述。这套体系的最终落实或许还需要一代人的努力，以及大量的资源、仁人志士的智慧以及上层的决心。

带教老师的体会

在住培轮转前，科里的住院医师都是专科医师，无论基本功、基本理论是否扎实，都对所在专科的技能（注意不是理论）有所求，也愿意学。但是现在科里都是轮转的住院医师，大多将来不从事这个专业，对这个专业的理论和技能都缺乏兴趣，就是浑浑噩噩地写病历、拉钩，待够时间后转到下一个专科。或许他们在一个专科踏踏实实干一年才能掌握相关专科技能，却要求他们每3个月转一个科室，还要掌握相关理论和技能，可能有点强人所难？

虽然有少数优秀的住院医师胸怀远大志向，但大多数住院医师的追求就是将来当个医生，没想成为医学大师。受限于天资、早年的教育基础和有效的激励，许多人确实没有能力从"大轮转"中收获预期的眼界和综合素质。

笔者认为，住培的本质目的是提高要求，如中学生一样，除了掌握基本的语文，还要求学习英语、文学、外国文学等。住培是医学本科教育的延伸。小学没打好基础，到了中学强行进实验班、兴趣班可能反而更加耽误了主课。

如果没有扎实的医学基础教育，即使到了各专科里也无法在规定的3个月里完成轮转要求，在自己所从事的专科领域又得不到充足的训练，得不偿失。扎实的基础教育，才能让住院医师在各个专科轮转中博采众长，为最终所从事的专科提供更宽阔的眼界和思路。

住院医师的体会

"草根"从来都不缺乏自嘲的方式，住院医师"民工"聊起自己的"搬砖"生活，吐槽有一万个段子，其中很大的共同点就是迷茫，有劲没处使，想学习不知道学什么、去哪里学。除了少数人得到高人指点或者机缘巧合，多数住院医师的规培就在迷茫中度过了。

有一个段子是：轮转3年导师都不认识自己，还问：你是谁的学生，什么都不会谁教的？让人啼笑皆非，细细想来，这或许是住院医师普遍迷茫的原因之一。常年在外轮转，既不能陪导师出门诊、替导师管患者，又不能做实验、出文章，师生的关系名存实亡。学生能主动找导师，亦或者导师能主动定期找学生的情况，又能有多少呢？

笔者认为，住院医师刚工作时都缺乏阅历和规划能力，正是需要导师指引的时候（不仅是学术上，更是生活乃至人生选择上）。轮转制度下，原有导师制的缺失或者不能落地，加重了年轻医生的迷茫。

去公司工作好歹有个上级领导，外企大都还有管理培训生，作为理应有制度优势的医疗培训体系，轮转和导师制不应冲突。

笔者的思考

总体来说，住培的本质和其他培训教育并无不同，都是牺牲眼前的效率和利益，换取将来更大的效率和利益。当这个"将来"有点远的时候，就好似一只驴子需要一根眼前的胡萝卜来鼓舞士气。现在的住院医师很清楚，需要每个阶段都有一根胡萝卜吃到嘴里才能继续前进；如果让住院医师觉得他付出了眼前的牺牲，却是别人享受将来的收益（哪怕仅仅是他觉得），那么住培往往也不能成功。

当然，落到操作层面，中国太辽阔，各级医院、各专业医生的培养方式各不相同，所面临的问题和困境也不同。一次讨论不可能解决所有问题，但能从各个角度引出问题和触发大家的思考和讨论总是好的。

一如商品经济的原始积累阶段都是一味扩大产能、产量，质量和个性化定制总是后期阶段的产物。笔者相信中国的住培体系会越来越好，但有的时候"螺旋式地上升"也是不可避免的。

主编导读（十三）

循规蹈矩还是创新突破——是什么困住了中国外科医生？

规则：是用来遵守的，还是打破的？

孟子说："不以规矩，不能成方圆。"这已经成为中国人代代相传的办事准则和方法学。

这个不难理解，规则本身是先人或者业界前辈经验和教训的总结，有了这些经验积累的总结，我们在工作中和日常生活中有据可循，会少走很多弯路，少办很多错事，也最大限度地避免了重复犯错的情况发生。

日常生活中遵守规则的必要性不胜枚举。我的一位飞行员朋友告诉我，在飞机起飞和降落前，会有一个近乎刻板的、机械性的三查七对，保证飞机状态和所有细节都被一一核准了，这样可以避免人为的差错。因为单单靠人的记忆和经验，总会有出错的概率。而在生命攸关的领域里，这种出错代价实在太大了。

我们马上会联想到医学领域，规则的重要性在这里被体现得更加淋漓尽致。在治疗疾病过程中，如果不按规则，自作主张、我行我素的话，那将分分钟付出生命的代价。在外科领域，这种对于规范的遵守不仅是对医院医疗制度的遵守，而且更加是体现在遵循前辈和同行所制定的行业指南、共识和规范上。如我们国内有肝癌诊治规范，是属于国家卫健委级别的指南，这个指南不断在更新，为国内的肝癌诊治带来标准化的指导，当然也是我们临床实践不可多得的宝典。

但从另一方面看，西方人常说：规矩是用来被打破的，中国人说：不破不立。

在我刚刚开始做外科医生的时候，外科界有大医生大切口（big surgeon，big incision）的说法，就是大医生做大手术，切口必须开得足够大，这样视野才好，而直视下的视野是外科手术的关键。但是在今天看，腹腔镜技术已经被广泛应用，很多手术在微创下进行，大医生可能不再用大切口，潜在原则已经被彻底打破，而且打破得对。

现在年轻的医生已经习惯于术前刷手是用专用海绵刷刷两次，不会去质疑为什么会是这样，也不感兴趣原来的手术刷手方式。早年的时候，外科医生是先要把双手在酒精桶里浸泡5分钟，之后才是刷手的。这个传统的规矩已经被打破多时了，但是在国内为什么会被打破？节点在哪儿？据说单单是因为一批从西方学习回来的医生说："美国早就不泡酒精了。"所以，我们也不泡了。结果是正确的，因为切口感染率没有因此上升。

问题出来了：我能回忆起来的规则的打破，或者外科技术的主要创新，几乎都源自欧美等西方国家，来源于中国的极少。

我国有一个特点，就是把别人创新出来的技术和点子，拿回来加以发挥，并且常常能够做到极致，使"原产地"大为逊色。前不久在日本召开的国际腹腔镜肝脏手术大会上，我们能够很清楚地感受到中国大陆的医生应用腔镜超声刀切肝技术的高超程度，已经到了炉火纯青的地步，使得首先发明和使用超声刀的西方人大为震惊和羡慕。

我们这么聪明，为什么领头创新的基本上不是我们？我们出了什么问题了吗？

我有意在遵守规则和打破规则方面提出一个题目进行讨论，主要是想促进中国医生敢于打破常规、进行创新的精神。实际上遵守和打破规则两者并不矛盾，是一个辩证的关系，主要是要找对节点。希望通过这个讨论，鼓励年轻医生广开才路、脑洞大开，在遵守医疗原则的基础上发挥我们的创新精神，使以后越来越多的新方法和技术原产于中国，然后还在中国发挥到极致。

规则：遵守，还是打破？

周　杰

南方医科大学　南方医院　肝胆外科

规则，究竟是遵守，还是应该打破？

有规则就要遵守，这是常识。然而也有这样的说法：规则就是用来打破的，不破不立，只有勇于打破现有规则，才能在工作和生活中求新求变。

诚然，不合实际的规则必须被打破，从而建立新的、适合当前实际情况的规则。但是，笔者认为，绝大多数规则仍然是需要遵守的，尤其是医疗行业的规则，更应该被严格地遵守。

医疗领域的规则是众多权威的医生和医学相关从业人士经过多年的积累所总结出的成果，遵循规则，可提高诊治的效果和效率。诊疗的过程不仅是针对疾病，而是针对患者、家庭甚至社会。不能只看效果，还要考虑不良反应，以及是否侵犯了患者的权利。随着生物科学的不断发展，部分技术涉及伦理问题，要处理好这些问题，医务人员必须遵守有关规则。

记得在20世纪80年代初一个寒冷的冬夜，笔者在基层医院实习。值班半夜来了个车祸急诊患者，患者呈失血性休克状态，腹腔穿刺有不凝固血液，诊断为腹腔内出血，肝脾破裂，由于当时医院条件所限，仅查了血型就紧急送手术室行剖腹探查术。开腹后发现腹腔血不多，肝脾无破损，出血来自腹膜后，再探查，发现是右肾破裂。于是，连夜去请泌尿外科医生，经过焦急的台上等待，在切口暴露不佳、肌松不完全的情况下，极其困难地完成了右肾切除术。右肾的损伤极其严重：肾门的位置断裂！术后由我们实习医生进行尿管留置，导尿管一插入，酱油色的尿液汹涌而出！当时后悔的情绪潮水般地涌来：如术前下尿管，肾损伤的诊断就能明确，就不至于半夜在手术台上焦急地等待泌尿外科医生、耽误了宝贵的抢救时间，手术切口也不至于如此别扭……第二天，科主任听我汇报完整个过程后，说了一句入院要查三大常规，这是经过多少年、从多少失败的病例中总结出来的经验。这句话，至今仍深深地印在我脑海里。

理念永远比技术更重要。敬畏生命是医学人文思想最基本的要求，也是最重要的核心，是一名医务工作者应该具备的最基本素养，更是悲天悯人情怀及大爱的基石。我们不能随意拿患者的生命、健康去尝试新疗法。动辄就以打破规则为由，随心所欲地根据自己的专长、爱好甚至利益来决定患者的治疗方案，是蛮干，是不讲科学，也会给患者带来灾难。遵守行业规则是医疗行业的底线，打着挑战规则的旗号、借口，做违反规则的事，是为行业所不齿。

违反规则、导致不良后果的例子，在现实生活、工作中比比皆是。在早期，很多医院分科不细，普通外科常常涵盖了胃肠、肝胆胰、血管、甲状腺、乳腺外科等专业。有一位主要从事血管外科的医生给自己的亲戚做胃切除手术，行胃肠吻合时，想当然地认为用血管吻合的方法和缝线会更完美。殊不知，胃的黏膜下血管极为丰富，当时的血管吻合用线过于滑润，未做黏膜下血管缝扎、又不锁边的外翻连续缝合很难达到止血的效果。结果，手术后患者出现吻合口活动性出血，不得已再次进行手术止血。近期也有医院因不遵守院内感染管理制度，导致69名患者感染丙肝病毒的重大医疗事件。

好规则固然不可或缺，让医护人员守规则更重要。我们既要建立科学合理的诊疗规则，更要培育医护人员的规则意识。打破规则谈何容易！规则不是谁都能打破的，大部分说这句话给自己行为背书的人，其实根本没有打破规则的资格与能力。作为普通人，还是好好遵守规则吧！如果人人都遵守规则，这个行业、这个世界就已经非常美好了。

规则的建立，都是出于一定的目的。随着发展，有的规则由于当初的局限性或许已经不再适合了，这时候才能去修正、打破它。当然规则也不是随便就能打破，一定要经过深思熟虑后才能作出选择，有了相当的新发现、新证据，才能修改规则。肝癌肝移植标准的修订，就是合理打破规则的典范。

肝癌肝移植最早遵循的是米兰标准。然而，在临床实践过程中发现：严苛的标准将相当多的患者拒之门外，使他们失去了移植（根治）的机会，但实际上这些患者仍然有很好的术后生存率。肝移植临床医生面临这样一个窘境：可能浪费一个供肝给了最终要复发的肝癌患者，也可能剥夺了一个原本可以治愈的肝癌患者获得供肝的权利，这两者实际上都是一种过失。学者们在米兰标准的基础上进行了科学的探索，尤其在中国大陆。中国是肝癌大国，肝癌人群基数庞大，大多数肝癌与乙肝肝硬化相关，且患者诊断时大多已经属于中晚期，常规肝切除的切除率低而复发率高，肝移植可能是他们唯一的希望。中国学者根据上述实际情况，在大量临床数据的基础上提出了符合中国国情的上海标准和杭州标准，这些标准超越并安全地扩展了米兰标准，使得更多的肝癌患者能接受肝移植治疗，且取得了和符合米兰标准患者相似的长期生存率。

所以，事物唯一不变的就是变化本身。如果现有的规则确实不合情理，那我们应该用合规的方法，来改变这个规则。打破规则的目的是跳出思维局限、推陈出新，从而建立更好的规则。遵守规则是挑战规则的前提，挑战规则是为了建立更好的规则，而新的规则又将面临新的挑战。

机体是脆弱的，治疗应该是温和的，尤其是有创的治疗，不应该造成额外的伤害。患病的机体就好像在荒芜冬月，死气沉沉，毫无生气。而适宜的治疗就恰似一场期待已久的春雨，温润了一切。我们面对的是一个个鲜活的生命，手术刀的轻，承载着生命的重。作为一名医生，尤其是外科医生，想要风平浪静、平平安安地度过每一天，真的太难。遵循规则，患者安好，你也安好，便是晴天。

参考文献

[1] Wang H, Zeng Y. Principles and rules: boundary and support for medical human-ity. Chin J Med Edu Res 2018; 17: 978-81.

[2] Zhang L, Zeng Y. Reverence for life: the cornerstone for medical humanity. Chin J Med Edu Res 2018; 17: 974-7.

[3] People's Daily Online. 69 patients in Jiangsu Dongtai People's Hospital were infected with hepatitis C virus, and the dean was removed from office. Available online: http://society.people.com.cn/n1/2019/0527/c1008-31104554.html

[4] Mazzaferro V, Regalia E, Doci R, et al. Liver transplantation for the treatment of small hepatocellular carcinomas in patients with cirrhosis. N Engl J Med 1996; 334: 693-99.

[5] Marsh JW, Dvorchik I, Iwatsuki S. Liver transplantation in the treatment of hepa-tocellular carcinoma. J Hepatobiliary Pancreat Surg 1998; 5: 24-8.

[6] Fan J, Zhou J, Xu Y, et al. Indication of liver transplantation for hepatocellu-lar carcinoma: Shanghai Fudan Criteria. Zhonghua Yi Xue Za Zhi 2006; 86: 1227-31.

[7] Zheng SS, Xu X, Wu J, et al. Liver transplantation for hepatocellular carcinoma: Hangzhou experiences. Transplantation 2008; 85: 1726-32.

Rules: abide or abandon?

Zhou Jie

Division of Hepatobiliopancreatic Surgery, Department of General Surgery, Nanfang Hospital, Southern Medical University, Guangzhou, China

Should we follow the rules or break them?

It is common sense that we must follow the rules. However, there is also such a saying that "rules are set to break". Only by daring to break the existing rules can we seek innovation and change in our life and work.

Indeed, unreasonable rules must be abandoned to establish new rules that fit realistic situations. However, most rules are properly established; thus, they must be obeyed. In particular, rules in the medical field should be strictly obeyed.

Medical guidelines are the summation of many authoritative medical practitioners after years of clinical practice and practice. Following medical guidelines can improve the efficiency and efficacy of diagnosis and treatment [1]. Proper diagnosis and treatment are not only relevant for specific diseases but also important for patients, families, and even society. Doctors should not only focus on the outcome but also consider the side effects, adverse reactions, and lawful rights of patients. As biological sciences develop, innovative research usually encounters ethical issues; thus, medical practitioners must follow the relevant standards to properly address these ethical issues.

It was a cold winter night in the early 1980s, and I was an intern in a local hospital. On my duty shift, there was a car accident in the middle of the night. The patient was in hemorrhagic shock, with massive non-clotting bloody ascites drawn from abdominal paracentesis. The initial diagnosis was "intra-abdominal bleeding, liver, and spleen rupture". Due to the limited resources of the local hospital at that time, the patient was rushed to the operating room for emergency exploratory laparotomy after only checking his blood type. When we opened his abdomen, we found that there was little leaking blood in the abdominal cavity, and the liver and spleen were intact. The bleeding actually came from the retroperitoneum. Further exploration eventually revealed that the right kidney rupture as the bleeding source. Therefore, we had to wait at the operating table for support from a urological surgeon. Due to the poor surgical view from an inappropriate incision and insufficient muscle relaxation, right nephrectomy was an extremely challenging operation to perform. Moreover, the right kidney was severely damaged as the renal hilum was lacerated. After the operation, as the intern, I was routinely responsible for placing a ureteral catheter. Once the catheter was placed, cola-colored urine was expelled. I was immediately overwhelmed by regrets; if I had placed the ureteral catheter before surgery, then the kidney injury would have been correctly diagnosed, thereby saving valuable time for the appropriate surgical incision to have been made and the urologist to arrive sooner. The next day, after hearing me recount the story, the chief of our department said: "the experience that we drew upon from many years and failed cases was that we should routinely perform blood, urine, and stool tests after hospital admissions". After decades, his words are still engraved deeply in my mind.

Virtue is far more precious than dexterity. The fundamental requirement of medical workers and the core of medical humanist education are awe of life [2]. Doctors must not jeopardize the health or lives of patients to test new therapies. Justifying untested methods as "revolutionary" and arbitrarily deciding the patient's treatment plan according to one's own experiences, preferences, or even interests is cruel, and could result in a disaster if the decision disobeys scientific principles. The bottom line of the medical industry is to follow the rules; thus, sacrificing patients' wellbeing to simply challenge the rules is strongly discouraged.

Examples of adverse consequences caused by violating rules abound in real life. In the early days, many hospitals did not set up sub-specialties in their departments, and "general surgery" often covered gastrointestinal, hepatobiliary, pancreatic, vascular, thyroid, breast surgery, and other specialties. At one time, a doctor who specialized in vascular surgery and performed a gastrectomy for one of his relatives. He assumed that the method and thread for vascular anastomosis was the best and applied these methods for gastrointestinal anastomosis. However, he did not realize that the submucosal layer of the stomach contained abundant blood vessels. To stop the bleeding, submucosal blood vessels should be ligated followed by continuous locking sutures. Additionally, the vascular thread was too smooth to ligate tightly. As a result, the patient experienced active bleeding from the gastrointestinal anastomosis after the operation and had to undergo another operation to stop the bleeding. Severe medical incidents as a result of rule violations still persist in the modern era. One hospital failed to follow management protocols for nosocomial infection causing 69 patients to be infected with hepatitis C [3].

While it is necessary to instate reliable rules, ensuring that people follow the rules is more critical. We should not only formulate scientific diagnosis and treatment guidelines but also foster the compliance of medical staff. Not everyone is capable of challenging medical guidelines. Some people may eschew guidelines to justify their mishandled medical behaviors; in fact, these individuals often do not have the qualifications or abilities to challenge these guidelines at all. If every medical worker abides by the rules, then the standards of the medical industry will improve.

Rules are established for certain purposes. As time passes, some rules may no longer be suitable and thus should be amended. Of course, these revisions should not be arbitrarily made, and instead should only be modified after careful consideration of recent discoveries and evidence. The revision of the criteria for liver cancer transplantation exemplifies this condition.

The "Milan criteria" was the earliest rule for liver transplantation to treat liver cancer [4]. However, in clinical practice, although a considerable number of patients had a good postoperative survival rate [5], they were rejected for liver transplantation by this strict standard and thus lost their opportunity for a radical cure. Liver transplantation faces the following dilemma: "wasting" a donor liver on a patient whose liver cancer may relapse or rejecting a liver versus a cancer patient who may be cured by a donated liver. Either direction would be a loss. Therefore, scholars began studying liver transplantation based on the Milan criteria in mainland China. China has a large population of patients with liver cancer, mostly due to hepatitis B cirrhosis. Many patients are already in the middle or late stages of liver cancer at the time of diagnosis, so conventional liver resection is hindered by a low complete resection rate and a high recurrence rate. Liver transplantation may be these patients' only hope. In this context, Chinese scholars proposed the "Shanghai criteria" and "Hangzhou criteria" based on evidence from a substantial amount of clinical data and research [6,7]. These new standards safely expanded the Milan criteria and allowed more liver cancer patients to receive liver transplants at a long-term survival rate similar to that of patients who meet the Milan criteria.

If pre-existing rules are unsuitable, then we should modify the rules to some degree. The intention of breaking the rules is to go beyond the existing boundaries of thinking and to bring forth new concepts to

守在生命的边缘
医者沉思录

establish better rules. Being able to follow the rules is the premise of revising rules, and the new rules will also face future challenges.

The human body is fragile, so treatment, especially of the invasive kind, should be moderated and not cause additional harm. The scalpel is light but carries the weight of life. As a doctor, and especially as a surgeon, our daily routine is restless and thus it is difficult to maintain a harmonious balance. Above all, better outcomes for patients can ensured by abiding by the rules.

References

［1］ Wang H, Zeng Y. Principles and rules: boundary and support for medical humanity. Chin J Med Edu Res 2018; 17: 978-81.

［2］ Zhang L, Zeng Y. Reverence for life: the cornerstone for medical humanity. Chin J Med Edu Res 2018; 17: 974-7.

［3］ People's Daily Online. 69 patients in Jiangsu Dongtai People's Hospital were infected with hepatitis C virus, and the dean was removed from office. Available online: http://society.people.com.cn/n1/2019/0527/c1008-31104554.html

［4］ Mazzaferro V, Regalia E, Doci R, et al. Liver transplantation for the treatment of small hepatocellular carcinomas in patients with cirrhosis. N Engl J Med 1996; 334: 693-99.

［5］ Marsh JW, Dvorchik I, Iwatsuki S. Liver transplantation in the treatment of hepatocellular carcinoma. J Hepatobiliary Pancreat Surg 1998; 5: 24-8.

［6］ Fan J, Zhou J, Xu Y, et al. Indication of liver transplantation for hepatocellular carcinoma: Shanghai Fudan Criteria. Zhonghua Yi Xue Za Zhi 2006; 86: 1227-31.

［7］ Zheng SS, Xu X, Wu J, et al. Liver transplantation for hepatocellular carcinoma: Hangzhou experiences. Transplantation 2008; 85: 1726-32.

主编导读（十四）

创新性临床研究中不可忽视的问题

医学技术创新应该需要伦理的约束。

我们目前正处于一个医学科技高速发展的年代，不时有令人惊喜的新技术、新发明诞生，有些技术确实为患者带来了良好的治疗效果。这些新技术爆发的现象不仅存在于外科领域里，如各种新的手术方式，包括联合肝脏离断及门脉结扎的分次肝切除手术（associating liver partition and portal vein ligation for staged hepatectomy，ALPPS）、腹腔镜下的复杂病例手术和机器人辅助的手术形式等；而且这些新技术还涵盖医学的各个领域，如靶向治疗药和免疫检查点抑制剂的应用及推广。它们给患者带来了切实的好处，有些原来难以治愈的疾病，如进展期肝癌，联合应用这些新技术、新措施以后，部分晚期肝癌患者经过治疗后得以转规/降期，有的还可以进行外科手术切除，大大提高了生存率，改善了生活质量，这肯定是一件好事。

但是如果让这些新技术无序发展、盲目繁衍，会带来新的问题。有些新技术和新药，对某些疾病适应证尚未被证实，就进行超适应证用药并且被广泛推广，虽然主观意愿是好的，但是存在客观的风险；而那些新的手术方式，如机器人辅助手术，由于需要严格的术前训练和经过学习曲线过程，在没有充分培训情况下，匆匆"上马"，常常会给患者带来更多的并发症和痛苦。

近期国内外作者的两则报道提示，腹腔镜胰十二指肠切除术的并发症发生率还是偏高的，只有当术者的腹腔镜操作例数达到或超过250例的时候，其并发症发生率才和传统开腹胰十二指肠切除术相接近，所以这些都要引起我们的广泛重视。

HBSN杂志曾经发表过一篇论述，讨论我们怎么来平衡外科新技术的开展和不损害患者利益的关系，一方面新技术一定要开展，不然医学科技永远不会进步（而且以后要争取更多的原创技术在国内启动）；另一方面，作为那些首先被安排施行新技术的患者，他们的健康安全和医疗利益应该被良好地保护，尽量不受伤害。当时这篇文章引发了非常大的反响，很多医务人员在线上、线下进行了热烈的讨论，虽然最后并没有定论，但是讨论本身就有很大的收获。

其中南京鼓楼医院外科专家仇毓东教授就提出了个人看法，他认为我们不能仅从医学人性和技术上来平衡和约束这两者的关系，更要从伦理学上进行规范。确实，从现代医学诞生这一刻起，就伴随着医学伦理学的发展，我们当然需要进一步从伦理学上去规范医疗新技术和患者安全健康的关系，而且要从伦理上进行约束。仇教授目前正好负责他们医院伦理学方面的工作，他主动请缨为我们HBSN杂志写下一篇医疗创新与伦理关系的述评。

我希望大家对此展开深入的讨论，并提出各种意见和建议。我个人深深地认为一种自由、活跃的氛围和思想是科学、艺术、文学和音乐创新的基本土壤。

创新性临床研究中的伦理问题

仇毓东

南京大学医学院附属鼓楼医院　医学伦理委员会

当今世界，医学科学领域迎来了飞速发展的时代，大量创新性的药物、器械、技术和诊疗方法不断涌现，给人类健康带来了巨大的获益。但是，在上述创新研发过程中往往孕育着潜在的风险，有的甚至危害到受试者的健康和生命。因此，医学伦理在创新性临床研究中扮演着越来越重要的角色，它好比在高速行驶的运载工具中发挥着刹车的作用。本文将在以下几个方面，阐述当今创新性临床研究中常见的医学问题和解决方案。

医学伦理的发展和原则

伦理（ethics）一词起源于希腊文ethos，品格、人格。伦理学是一门研究人在道德领域价值的学科，而医学伦理学关注和研究的是医生在行医过程中应该遵循的道德规范。

古希腊时期，医学之父Hippocrates提出了"无损于患者为先"的伦理标准，成为千百年来行医者需要恪守的道德规范。但另一方面，医学技术的发展需要持续性探索和创新，同样也是一个不断试错的过程，这就给患者带来了风险和痛苦，如何平衡好临床研究中的受益和风险是医务工作者长期以来面临的难题。

为了获得更多、更准确的医学知识，学者们长期以来作了不懈的努力。古罗马著名医生Claudius Galenus，通过动物解剖发现了许多与人体相似的解剖学结构，大大推动了解剖学的发展，但同时也出现了许多错误。

文艺复兴时期的许多科学巨匠质疑了Galenus以及许多前辈的观

点，但由于宗教的束缚无法在公开场合展示他们从尸体解剖上获得的新知识和新理论。经过漫长的探索和斗争，人们逐渐意识到基于宗教的传统伦理观念阻碍了科学的发展。可是，新的医学伦理又将如何确立呢？

为此，人类还要经过百余年的摸索，并付出沉重的代价。我们耳熟能详的许多医学史上重大发现的都背负着巨大的伦理阴影。人类历史上率先揭示胃消化功能的William Beaumont（1785－1853），就是在一位不幸腹部受伤的患者Alexis St Martin承受了8年未予治疗的胃外瘘痛苦的基础上获得的成果。

美国外科医生J. Marion Sims（1813－1883）为了探索膀胱－阴道瘘的治疗方法，长期在黑人妇女身上做手术试验，使这些受试者身心承受了巨大的痛苦。牛痘疫苗的发明者英国人E. Jenner，为了验证其疫苗的有效性，不惜以孩子作为试验者；Jenner牺牲了医学伦理，拯救了英国数十万天花患者，而且最终让全人类获益。

在当时的社会条件下，Sims和Jenner均被广为称颂，没有人质疑他们在研究过程中为受试者带来的伤害，更没有人关心受试者所承受的身心摧残。上述事态到第二次世界大战发展最严重，纳粹分子用犹太人做活体解剖，日本侵略者用中国人做细菌实验都严重违背了人类的道德底线。

但奇怪的是，这些人在审判战犯的法庭上拒不认罪，声称他们的行为是科学研究，虽然损害了某些个体的权益，但研究成果却可以使全人类获益。经过激烈的法庭辩论，最终这些法西斯分子被判决犯下反人类罪行，得到了应有的惩罚。

长达数年的法庭辩论，促使法律界、医学界进行了全面、深刻的反思，催生了人类历史上第一部有关人体研究的国际伦理指南——《纽伦堡法典》。其中特别强调了对接受人体研究的受试者个人的保护，该法典为人体研究的伦理原则奠定了法律基础。

但遗憾的是，20世纪40～60年代，违反伦理原则，触及道德底线，尤其是为了商业利益危害受试者权益的临床研究时有报道，其中最为严重的就是塔斯基吉研究（The Tuskegee Study）实验。399名感染梅毒的黑人在不知情的情况下没有被实施任何治疗，放任疾病发展直至悲惨地死去。

对此，有良知的医生Henry K. Beecher在《新英格兰医学杂志》上发表了题为《伦理与临床研究》（*ethics and clinical research*）一文，明确指出临床研究的伦理要素：①知情同意，充分告知，尊重患者（受试者）的选择；②凭良心做事，做一名富于同情心、负责的研究者；③研究伦理属性取决于开始，结果合理不证明手段合理；④发表以不符合伦理手段获得的数据是不可接受的。

此后，揭露塔斯基吉研究的贝尔蒙报告相继出台，提议建立伦理审查制度，为美国联邦法规《保护受试者》（45CFRPart46 "Common Rule"）的编撰奠定了基础。

1964年，世界医学会（the World Medical Association，WMA）在赫尔辛基的第八次大会上通过此宣言，关键内容包括：将动物实验和实验室数据，以及临床研究方案、提交给一个独立的伦理委员会审核。对患者权益的关注应超出对科学和社会利益的关注，保护隐私；确认危险超出潜在获益时，应暂停研究，由受试者自愿并作出书面知情同意，受试者无法作出时由其法定代理人同意；如果免签知情同意，应提交给独立的委员会；每个患者，包括对照组的患者，都应确保予以最佳的诊断和治疗；措施违反本宣言原则的研究、报告不应予以发表。至此，临床研究中的伦理原则得到了根本的确立。

临床研究方法的进展

临床医学的进步离不开临床研究，医学从诞生至今经历了漫长的经验医学时代，此时的临床研究仅停留在医生个人经验的总结。"神农氏勇尝百草"可能是人类最早的临床药物试验，随着现代自然科学的发展，医学也进入崭新的时代。

20世纪中叶，临床医学迈入基于证据的循证医学时代。证据的等级成为临床决策的决定性依据，处在金字塔顶端的是多中心、随机对照研究得出的结果。

在新药研发领域，1990年成立的人用药品技术要求国际协调理事会（The International Conference on Harmonization of Technical Requirements for Registration of Pharmaceuticals for Human Use，ICH），该国际组织将监管机构和制药行业聚集在一起，讨论药品的科学和技术问题并制定指导原则。

2017年，我国国家药品监督管理总局成为ICH的正式成员，我国也相继制定并颁布了《药物临床试验质量管理规范》（Good Clinical Practice，GCP），进一步规范了药物上市前的临床研究。

仔细研读国内外药物临床试验所遵循的科学原则，我们能发现其主要的依据还是基于循证医学的证据等级。进入21世纪00年代，医学迅速迈入了精准医学时代。

而追求个体化、精准诊疗的精准医学对临床研究提出了更高的要求和挑战。许多极富创新性的精准诊疗策略由于多种限制（主要是无法获得满足循证医学要求的研究和对照组病例数）无法获得足够高等级的证据。

因此，新的临床研究策略应运而生。2017年，《新英格兰医学》发表了文章《临床路径的变迁——实用性试验》（*the changing face of clinical trails—Pragmatic Trails*）提出，外来的临床研究将从单纯注重证据的实证性研究转向同时兼顾科学性、有效性、安全性和成本－效益的实效性研究，从而开启了临床研究的创新天地。

创新性研究中的伦理问题

在众多的临床研究中，外科技术的探索和发展具有其独特性。由于存在高风险、高难度和高度技术依赖性，外科的临床研究无法严格遵循GCP为基础的临床研究策略。为此，牛津大学发起并创立了外科医生、临床流行病学家、统计学家和学术编辑等组成的IDEAL（Idea Development Exploration Assessment and Long-term follow up，IDEAL）协作网。

作为国际性的外科创新学术组织，其成员包括来自全球的相关研究人员。经过不断实践，研究者发现IDEAL研究模式，不仅在外科技领域有广泛的应用，还可以拓展至更富有创新性的治疗策略和方法的研发和推广。其循序渐进，逐步提升的理念完全符合当前实效性研究的思路。

所谓IDEAL，主体部分分为五个阶段：设计、开发、探索、评价，长期随访。分别采用不同的临床设计，逐渐增加病例数，提高证据等级，夯实科学基础。在创新性研究中，除了上述临床研究模式外，还特别重视前期阶段，也就是基础研究、临床前研究等，将体外实验、动物实验、材料和器械等结果和信息融合到整体研究过程中。

在进行每一步临床试验前，都要求经过严格的伦理审查，最大限度地保障受试者安全和权益。同时，为了公开研究过程，还要求研究者对各阶段的研究设计登记注册，以维护研究的公平、公正，也间接保护了研究者的权益。在IDEAL理念的指导下，近年来大量创新性医学研究成果不断涌现，极大地推动了健康事业的繁荣和发展。

当今医学已进入了创新发展的时代，而随着社会文明的进步，医学伦理问题显得更加重要。我们每一位临床医生和研究者在拓展自己的研究领域、开创新的临床技术、解决复杂的临床问题时更应该牢记伦理原则，这样才能使我们的患者得到更有效的治疗，使医学科学获得健康光明的前途。

参考文献

［1］Ford I, Norrie J. Pragmatic Trials. N Engl J Med 2016; 375: 454-63.

［2］McCulloch P, Feinberg J, Philippou Y, et al. Progress in clinical research in surgery and IDEAL. Lancet 2018; 392: 88-94.

［3］Garas G, Cingolani I, Patel V, et al. Surgical Innovation in the Era of Global Surgery: A Network Analysis. Ann Surg 2020; 271: 868-74.

［4］Rogers WA, Hutchison K, McNair A. Ethical Issues Across the IDEAL Stages of Surgical Innovation. Ann Surg 2019; 269: 229-33.

［5］Dimick JB, Sedrakyan A, McCulloch P. The IDEAL Framework for Evaluating Surgical Innovation: How It Can Be Used to Improve the Quality of Evidence. JAMA Surg 2019; 154: 685-6.

［6］Bilbro NA, Hirst A, Paez A, et al. The IDEAL Reporting Guidelines: A Delphi Consensus Statement Stage Specific Recommendations for Reporting the Evaluation of Surgical Innovation. Ann Surg 2021; 273: 82-5.

守在生命的边缘
医者沉思录

Ethical issues in innovative clinical research

Qiu Yudong

Medical Ethics Committee, the Affiliated Drum Tower Hospital of Medical School of Nanjing University, Nanjing, China

In today's world, medical science has entered an era of rapid development. Numerous new drugs, devices, technologies, and diagnosis and treatment methods continue to emerge, bringing great benefits to our human health. However, there are potential risks in the above innovative research and development process, and some can even endanger the health or life of the test subjects. As a result, medical ethics plays an increasingly important role during the rapid development of innovative clinical research, acting as a "brake" on this high-speed vehicle. This article will illustrate some medical problems and solutions that are common in today's clinical research in the following aspects.

Development and principles of medical ethics

The word ethics originates from the Greek "*ethos*", which means character/personality. Ethics is a subject that studies the value of human beings within the scope of morality, while medical ethics concerns the moral norms that doctors should follow in the process of practicing medicine. In the ancient Greek period, Hippocrates, the father of medicine, proposed the ethical standard of doctors, "first do no harm to the patient", which has become a moral code that practitioners need to abide by for thousands of years. On the other hand, the development of medical technology requires continuous exploration and innovation, which is a process of "trial and error", bringing potential risks and pain to patients. How to balance the "benefit" and "risk" is a long-standing problem faced by medical workers.

Many of the great discoveries in the history of medicine that we are familiar with bear huge ethical shadows. William Beaumont (1785—1853) is the first person who revealed the digestive function of the stomach, but he obtained his finding from Alexis St. Martin, a patient who suffered from an untreated external gastric fistula for 8 years after his abdominal injury. The American surgeon J. Marion Sims (1813—1883), conducted long-term surgical experiments on black women to explore the treatment of vesicovaginal fistula, causing them to suffer tremendous physical and mental torture. Years of court debates have led to a comprehensive and profound reflection in the legal and medical circles, in which the Nuremberg Code came into being. As the first international ethical guide on clinical research in history, the Nuremberg Code particularly emphasizes the protection of patient volunteers who undergo clinical research. The Code lays a legal foundation for the ethical principles of clinical research.

In this regard, Henry K. Beecher published an article "ethics and clinical research" in *The New England Journal of Medicine*, which stated the ethical requirements of clinical research: (I) informed consent: fully informed and respect the choice of the patient (subject); (II) researchers with responsibility, compassion and conscience improve the reliability of research outcome; (III) the ethical attributes of research depend on the inception, the results do not justify means; (IV) whether to publish data obtained by unethical means is arguable. These statements established a solid foundation for 45 CFR Subpart A (the Common Rule), which is a compilation of the US Federal Regulations to protect research subjects. In 1964, the World Medical Association (WMA) adopted this declaration at its eighth congress in Helsinki. The Common Rule stated that all animal experiments, laboratory data, and research protocols should be submitted to institutional review boards (IRB) for preview. Patient rights and privacy should override societal and scientific interests and research should be suspended when risks outweigh potential benefits. Informed consent should be signed by the research subject or the subject's legally authorized representative, and exceptions should be reviewed by the IRB. Each patient, including those in the control group, should be assured of optimal treatment. Research should not be published if its measures violate the principles of this declaration. Thus far, the ethical principles in clinical research were preliminarily established.

The development of clinical research methods

Early clinical studies were merely summaries of physicians' personal experiences. "Shennong's courage to taste hundreds of herbs" may be the earliest clinical drug test in human history. With the development of modern natural science, clinical medicine has transitioned into evidence-based medicine since the middle of the last century. The level of evidence becomes the decisive basis for the clinical decision-making process, and the top-level evidence is from multicenter, randomized, controlled studies.

In the field of new drug development, there is the International Conference on Harmonization of Technical Requirements for Registration of Pharmaceuticals for Human Use (ICH). The ICH, established in 1990, is an organization that brings together regulatory agencies and the pharmaceutical industry to discuss the scientific and technical issues of drugs and formulate guidelines. In 2017, the Food and Drug Administration of China officially joined ICH and China subsequently published the "Good Clinical Practice (GCP)", which strengthened the regulation of clinical research before drug marketing. The scientific principles followed by drug clinical trials globally mainly depended on evidence-based medicine. In 2017, an article named "the changing face of clinical trials—pragmatic trials" was published in *The New England Journal of Medicine*, suggesting that clinical research should shift from evidential trials, which primarily focus on evidence-based research, to pragmatic trials, which concurrently take science, safety, and cost-effectiveness into account [1]. This article opened a new world of clinical research facing to the era of precision medicine and innovation.

Ethical issues in innovative research

In many clinical studies, the development path of surgical techniques has its uniqueness. The surgical operation usually involves high risk, high difficulty, and is highly technology dependent, clinical research in the surgical field cannot strictly follow the GCP-based research guidelines. Therefore, Oxford University started up the IDEAL Collaboration (Idea, Development, Exploration, Assessment, and Long-term follow-up), which consists of surgeons, clinical epidemiologists, statisticians, and academic editors. As a global surgical innovative academic organization, the IDEAL Collaboration has researchers from all over the world [2]. Through countless practices, researchers found that the IDEAL research mode is not only applicable to surgical technology but also can be extended to improve new treatment plans. Its recommendation to have different plans at each stage is completely in line with the current thinking of pragmatic trials.

The so-called IDEAL divides research into five stages: idea, development, exploration, assessment, and long-term follow-up. As the research continues, researchers gradually increase the number of cases, improve the level of evidence, and consolidate the research background by adopting different clinical designs [3]. In innovative research, besides the clinical research mode mentioned above, a pre-ideal stage is also very substantial. Pre-ideal stage integrates the results of preclinical research, including in vitro experiments, animal experiments, and results from mechanical and material science into the overall clinical research. Strict ethical review is required to ensure the safety and interests of subjects to the maximum extent before each step of clinical trials [4]. To disclose the research process, researchers are required to register their research designs at all stages to maintain the impartiality of the research, which simultaneously protects the rights and interests of researchers [5]. Under the guidance of the IDEAL Collaboration in recent years, numerous innovative medical research findings combined, which greatly promoted the development and prosperity of the medical health field [6].

Medicine today is in a stage of rapid development. With the continued development of our social civilization, medical ethical issues become more prominent. Every clinician and researcher should keep ethical principles in mind when pursuing their research fields, discovering new clinical technologies, and solving complicated clinical problems. By doing so, our patients can be treated fairly and effectively, so that our medical science will carry a healthy and bright future.

References

［1］Ford I, Norrie J. Pragmatic Trials. N Engl J Med 2016; 375: 454-63.

［2］McCulloch P, Feinberg J, Philippou Y, et al. Progress in clinical research in surgery and IDEAL. Lancet 2018; 392: 88-94.

［3］Garas G, Cingolani I, Patel V, et al. Surgical Innovation in the Era of Global Surgery: A Network Analysis. Ann Surg 2020; 271: 868-74.

［4］Rogers WA, Hutchison K, McNair A. Ethical Issues Across the IDEAL Stages of Surgical Innovation. Ann Surg 2019; 269: 229-33.

［5］Dimick JB, Sedrakyan A, McCulloch P. The IDEAL Framework for Evaluating Surgical Innovation: How It Can Be Used to Improve the Quality of Evidence. JAMA Surg 2019; 154: 685-6.

［6］Bilbro NA, Hirst A, Paez A, et al. The IDEAL Reporting Guidelines: A Delphi Consensus Statement Stage Specific Recommendations for Reporting the Evaluation of Surgical Innovation. Ann Surg 2021; 273: 82-5.

主编导读（十五）

如何解决患者入院前、出院后服务的难题？

我们现有的医疗服务体系实际上并不包括患者入院前和出院后的照顾。我们时常看到很多住院前的患者（大部分是外地患者）在完成门诊检查和评估、开具住院证明以后，不得不在医院附近的小旅馆里等候。

实际上有些患者是需要进行一些手术前的输液和调理的，但是这在院外不可能实现，患者常常像热锅上的蚂蚁似的一天天在焦虑和不安中等待医院召唤。此时，没有一个简单的医疗机构或者实体能够给予其照顾，帮助联系或者通知安排住院路径等。

同样地，在手术后，由于大医院的床位利用率问题，会让患者尽快出院。有的医院采用快速康复理念后，早出院就成为象征患者早康复的指标。当然这没有错，但是患者出院后直接面临着没有相应的医疗机构接手照顾的问题，患者在出院后会有无助感和不安全感。

加上万一真有些什么事情，在大医院再次挂号都非常困难；有些外地患者在出院的当口不便于长途旅行，不得不重新回到入院前住的"小旅馆"里面过渡。所以我们常常会面临患者不愿意出院，愿意在医院里再"养一养"的情况，实际上是为了获得一份安全感。

这个问题存在已久了，为什么会得不到改善呢？或者是不是实际上没有人努力去改善呢？在西方发达国家（不管是欧陆医疗系统、英联邦医疗系统还是北美医疗系统）会好一些，因为他们有地段医生和私人医生来接手。我接触的医疗卫生主管部门的人士，他们对于发达国家全程医疗管理系统并不是不知晓，反而是早就了如指掌了。

多年以前我国也曾经启动过全科医生体系，显然是一个努力的尝试。但是到如今，我们开展的全科医生是"光听到雷声"好几年，还是没有真正"下雨"。其中深层原因我们并不了解，反正尝试了半天，全程医疗照顾还是明显不足。近年来，为了均匀医疗资源分配，有些医院之间发展了"医联体"模式，此模式或许有些帮助，但是大都是个别的"自由恋爱"，也没有系统保证。

我有时在想，我们有庞大的医疗行政管理机构，又有强悍的总体调配体制，为什么就不建立（或者建不成）一套体系来解决对患者全程医疗管理的问题呢？另一边，目前很多民营的医疗单位，正在想尽一切办法从各方面"揾食"，为什么不建立一些院前、院后的医疗服务机构呢？这些机构对医疗专业的要求并不高，甚至可以把大医院周围专门给"外地患者"准备的小旅馆改成这种简单医疗场所（当然需要行医执照），来完成全程医疗管理中的一个环节。这些都是难解之谜。

当我同丁香园版主谈起这个话题，他同样非常感兴趣。作为非临床医务人员的版主从另外一个角度来看问题，我觉得也很有意思，不无道理，在此分享一二。

目前的问题还反映了当下医疗体系急功近利，注重"治疗"、不重视"管理"的困境。现存的已经流程化、标准化、制度化的诊疗流程中，保留情怀的一线医务人员在付出情怀时常常怀揣的是不安，收获的是"失去"，却无力改变这个现状。对于患者的院前、院后全程化管理，现有的临床资源还无法做到从患者角度出发、以人为本地全程化服务，不管是重症还是轻症。

医院的流程是让那些培养出来的优秀医生在院内尽量把看病做得完美无缺，院方简单直接地给出几个考核指标，科室管理者需要结合自己科室的现状进行调配，这个体系很难做到"除人类之病痛、助健康之完美"的理想信念。

所以本次我邀请了国内著名外科专家，世纪坛医院外科主任彭吉润教授，结合他自己的真实体会对这个问题进行了分析和阐述。我觉得这篇文章深入分析了院前、院后管理的刚需，现存体系下无法改变既定事实的无奈。也有对真正发达体系下患者应有就医体验的追寻、向上的追问与呼唤。

非常希望这个问题能够引起大家的共鸣和讨论。有识者也可以提出官方和民间的解决方案；当然也希望医疗行政部门能够筹划一些合理的方案来改善或者解决这个缺憾。实际上我们最大的共识是让我们国家的医疗体系真正覆盖医疗管理的全程，更好地为患者服务，共同创建一个温暖的、安全的、成熟的社会体系。

院外服务：急需建立和完善的社会体系

彭吉润[1, 2, 3]

[1]北京世纪坛医院　肝胆肿瘤外科
[2]北京大学第九临床医学院
[3]首都医科大学肿瘤医院

二十多年前，我父亲的好友因患胰腺癌，从家乡来北京看病。在北京某著名医院就诊后，等待住院手术。因为这家医院的床位十分紧俏，一般手术前一天，患者才能住进医院，所以患者和他的家人，只能暂时住在那家医院附近的一间地下室旅馆等待。

一天，他的夫人，一位退休的护士，打电话给我，说患者因为饮食不佳，十分虚弱，所以想请我帮忙，在我当时供职的医院开一些葡萄糖注射液以及生理盐水一类的液体，她拿回旅馆中，自己给患者输注。我自然是尽力帮忙，但我问她，为什么不在就诊的那家医院开这些呢，她回答说没有人会管这样的事；而且，她还不敢让主治医生知道，自己擅自做主，给患者做这些治疗，怕他们不高兴……

之后不久，患者的夫人告诉我，手术比较顺利，患者已经痊愈出院了。但最终的结果正像我们知道的那样，胰腺癌这种疾病极为险恶，预后很差，术后大约不到一年，患者就因肿瘤复发去世了。

那时，通过这件事，我就在想，这些外地来京手术的重病患者，真是不易，不但要在这座陌生的大都市中，自行找到心仪的医院、医生就诊，卑微而耐心地等待一张住院床位，而且住院前、后还要自行解决围手术期遇到的各种医疗问题。

上面这位患者的夫人恰巧曾做过几年护士，还可以做一些类似输液这样的治疗措施，可其他人遇到这样的问题该怎么办呢？何况，很多问题，即使你做过医生、护士，也是难以解决的。

二十多年过去了，胰腺癌的总体治疗效果，仍然令人悲观。而我们在住院前、后，为那些肿瘤患者、重病患者提供的院外基本医疗服务，比那时进步了吗？总体而言，在我看来，即使有所改善，改善的程度似乎也十分有限。近期我治疗的一个患者的经历，为这个负面判断又提供了一个佐证。

这是一个结肠癌合并肝脏转移的患者，他在北京周边一家省城的肿瘤专科医院进行了手术治疗，之后在那家医院的肿瘤内科进行了标准疗程的化疗。来找到我们的时候，肝脏上的肿瘤复发了，而且处理起来比较棘手。

我们问患者和家属，为什么化疗后很长时间没有再密切地随访观察，以致情况发展到这么糟糕的地步才来治疗呢？他们回答说，手术后，外科医生就把患者转给了肿瘤内科医生；而肿瘤内科医生做完化疗后，就再没有其他医生接手照看他们，也没有人后续再给予他们更详细的指导和帮助了。

上面这两个真实案例，其实反映了我们的医疗系统，特别是在手术相关科室，多年来存在的一个服务盲点或偏差，即我们将医疗工作的重点和资源，更多地聚焦在住院期间的诊疗服务上。

而对住院前、后的手术患者，特别是那些肿瘤和重病患者，不但住院前难以获得令人满意的医疗照顾和适当处理，而且这些患者一旦出院回到社区，鉴于相关疾病诊治的专业性很强，很多人因此就陷入了一种无人照看、不知如何进行后续治疗和随访的困境，而任由其自生自灭，更遑论还有人会进一步提供心理支持、财务指导、语言服务等更显奢侈的照护了（这些在西方发达国家的医疗中心，都是常规的服务项目）。

在内科领域，类似的问题也同样存在。这种现象背后所反映的是，即使是在中国最发达的类似北上广这样的中心都市中，仍然缺乏能真正发挥作用的院前、院后医疗服务体系，能够和住院医疗服务完美配套。

在我国，随着高铁的普及，以大都市为中心的 N 小时工作、生活圈逐渐形成，周边城镇与大城市之间的交通越来越便捷；同时，医疗保险异地报销渠道开通后，患者就医的选择性也大大增加了。

这两种因素相叠加，会使得越来越多的肿瘤患者、重病患者，集中到北上广这类医疗资源丰富的中心都市，寻求更为优质的医疗服务，从而会使得这些地方，住院医疗服务与院前、院后服务脱节这一问题显得更为突出，而寻求这一问题的解决办法，也显得尤为迫切。

目前，在我们这样一个以公立医疗系统为主的国家，各级医疗主管部门似乎对这个问题也没有足够的重视。他们为医院制定并施行的各种考评指标中，在某种程度上仅仅把患者——我们医疗体系的主要服务对象，当成了医疗环节中一个个患有不同病种的客观考核参照物，而对他们获得的住院医疗服务与院前、院后服务严重脱节这一问题，如果在诸多考核指标里其实是被考虑到了的话，也只有那项模棱两可的称为"患者满意度"的指标勉强可以用来敷衍一下。

在这种考评机制下，当院长、医务处、绩效考核部门以及科主任和带组医生们把主要精力都放在努力提高出院患者数、住院患者中手术病例的比例、代表医院和科室诊治疾病种类多寡的CMI值、大中型手术占比、微创手术占比，降低平均住院天数、药占比、耗材占比以及满足集采药物和耗材的完成率等种类繁杂的考核指标时，谁还有精力和心思去关心某个患者入院前有没有给予适当医疗照看、出院后伤口疼痛是否需要药物缓解、患者是否能按时随访这些看起来不怎么起眼的"小事"上呢？

公道地说，国内的医疗主管部门也正在努力建立更合理的医疗分级诊疗体系，试图让所有的患者都得到与其所患疾病相适合的、连续性的诊疗服务，无奈目前正在建立的这个系统，对解决上述问题，帮助不大。单单各家机构之间医疗信息系统不兼容这一项，就足以让各级各类医疗当事方望洋兴叹了，各级各类医疗机构所属部门之间的利益、条块分割，更是进一步限制了资源的整合和协同。

前一阵子，国内兴起了所谓的"医联体"，试图找到一种进行分级诊疗以及不同级别医院间相互转诊和协作的新路径，但真正实施起来，其实质更像是牵头的各大中心型或旗舰级医院之间在自由竞争和扩张其各自的势力范围。此外，牵头单位和"医联体"的其他组成单位之间看似形成了某种长期的一对多的伙伴关系，但并没有形成一种具有行政或法律约束力的机制进行保证，最终大多数"医联体"往往沦为了展示政绩的一种手段。

面对上述种种困难，这难道真是一道无解的难题吗？目前，中国的总体经济实力已经位居世界第二，具有无比庞大和强大执行力的医疗行政管理机构，更具有令世人惊叹的社会治理和管控体制，可以让百万级、千万级人口的城市在一夜之间静默下来，为什么不能借鉴新冠大流行期间所形成的多种协调机制和契机，在国家层面进行顶层设计，建立和完善一套真正有效运转的分级诊疗体系，来解决问题呢？

"他山之石，可以攻玉"。其他发达国家如东邻日本的以公立医院为主的医局系统，以澳大利亚、加拿大为代表的英联邦国家家庭医生、地区诊所与中心医院、专科医生之间的转诊系统，美国的医疗集团制度等，都早已在这个领域进行了多年的探索与实践，也积累了很多经验和教训，搭建了各式各样"过河的桥梁"，可供我们的医疗主管部门在进行制度设计时予以借鉴。

尽管各国的国情确实千差万别，即使在我们这个幅员辽阔的国家内部，各地区之间的经济发展水平以及医疗服务水平也不尽相同，但人类社会为患者服务的初心是相通的；凭借我们国家和社会目前的总体实力和条件，还以"摸着石头过河"为借口，一直站在河里，而不去架桥铺路，就有点儿说不过去了。

但无论最后采取哪些顶层设计和实施路径去解决问题，关键一点，一定要予以充足的经费投入。目前分级诊疗体系不那么成功的关键原因之一，就是我们对最基层医疗部门的投入远远不够，难以吸引相关人才全身心地投入基层医疗服务领域。基层医疗机构人才匮乏，收入低、地位低、能力欠缺，导致构成分级诊疗的基石难以稳固，也难以满足患者不断增长的各种医疗需求。

此外，对医院特别是大型、中心型医院而言，也应重视人性化医疗路径的设计和实践，主动为患者提供和对接配套的院前、院后服务项目和体系。当然，在进行顶层设计时，也应考虑投入经费用于对这些提供医疗服务的重要主体的补偿，比如，设立医保报销的收费项目，否则，让医院耗费大量资源提供太多的无偿服务，恐怕难以为继。

另一个可供探讨的选择是，不妨将院前、院后配套医疗服务业务这一远未被满足的需求，开放给民营机构进行探索性经营。近期在北京等大城市兴起的、颇受一些中产阶级患者欢迎的"陪诊"服务，其实就是这类探索性服务的一种萌芽。如果能将这类服务性业态逐步培育和完善起来，也许会为上述问题找到一条有效的市场化解决路径，至少，会为以公立医疗为主体的分级诊疗系统提供一种有效的补充。

无论是进行顶层设计，还是改善医疗路径的设计，都应该多倾听医疗服务一线人员——医生、护士和各类医疗辅助人员的意见和建议，广泛调研，谋定而后动，而不是依靠缺乏医疗一线实践经验的医政官员与相熟的专家在会议室里闭门造车。

离开了医疗一线人员的认可和支持，即使出发点再好的制度和设计，也难以真正获得成功。最令人担心的事情是，这个问题提出来以后，可能确实会得到相关医疗主管部门的关注和重视，但提出的解决方案，只是把问题简单地又制定为一项新的考核指标，把压力又平白无故地加到医院和一线医务人员头上。非常不幸的是，根据墨菲定律，每当有类似的担心时，我们从没有失望过。

而就我们医护人员方面而言，在一个理想的院前、院后服务体系建立起来之前，还是要提倡树立一种把自己经治的患者当成"我的患者"的理念，以科室、团队为单位，利用现代化的各种通信媒介如微信等，尽可能为那些肿瘤、重症患者，多提供一点额外的服务和指导，把患者尽可能地纳入全生命周期管理。尽管我们能做的有限，也只能照顾到少数患者，但也聊胜于无。

Peri-hospital care: time to have a system for arranging patient care before and after hospitalization

Peng Jirun[1,2,3]

[1] Department of Hepatobiliary Surgery, Beijing Shijitan Hospital, Capital Medical University, Beijing, China
[2] Ninth School of Clinical Medicine, Peking University, Beijing, China
[3] School of Oncology, Capital Medical University, Beijing, China

Twenty years ago, a friend of my father, suffering from pancreatic cancer, came to a famous hospital in Beijing from my hometown for surgery. While waiting for hospitalization, his wife, a retired nurse, came to me for help, saying her husband was very weak, and she wanted me to prescribe some take-home normal saline and glucose solution for patient infusion during their hotel stay. I did the favor, but asked her why not asking the doctors in that hospital to prescribe these drugs. She said that no one would care about such things. She didn't even dare to let the doctors in charge know that she would give patient these treatments without permission, which would irritate them.

Through this experience, I realized that, for patients, coming to Beijing for surgery is not easy. Not only do they have to wait humbly and patiently for a hospital bed in this unfamiliar city, but also deal with various medical problems before and after hospitalization. The above-mentioned patient's wife was a nurse and could handle treatments like infusions, but what about other people? Besides, many medical problems are difficult to solve even for a doctor or nurse.

Twenty years later, have we improved our basic out-of-hospital medical services for those with cancer and critically ill patients before and after hospitalization? To be fair, there has been some improvement, but the extent appears to be very limited. The ordeal of a patient with colon cancer and liver metastases who came to me for help provided evidence for this negative judgment. The patient had undergone surgery and a standard course of chemotherapy at a major oncology hospital in a provincial capital city. However, at discharge, he was given no further detailed medical guidance, and consequently he did not closely follow up his diseases. By the time he came to me, the liver tumor recurred and progressed to an intractable level.

These two examples shed light on a blind spot of our hospital system over the years: We have focused our efforts and resources on the diagnosis and treatment during hospitalization, while often fail to provide adequate medical care before and after hospitalization for patients, especially those with tumors or other severe diseases. Moreover, given the highly specialized professional knowledge required, many patients discharged back into the community were at the mercy of luck, as no one knows how to take care of them, and follow-up visits are often missed, not to mention the more advanced care of psychological support, financial guidance, language services, etc.

In China, with the development of the high-speed railway systems, travel between cities and towns is becoming ever more convenient. Cancer patients and seriously ill patients crowd into central cities such as Beijing and Shanghai to seek better medical services. In these places, the discontinuity between inpatient medical services and pre-hospital and post-hospital services is more prominent, so a solution to these problems is particularly imperative.

In current China, where public medical system is predominant,

守在生命的边缘
医者沉思录

medical authorities do not seem to pay enough attention to this issue. Among the many indicators that they laid down for hospital evaluations, perhaps only one of them labeled as "patient satisfaction" implicitly touches on a hospital's ability to solve this problem. Under this evaluation system, presidents and department chairs of large and medium-sized hospitals are pressured to focus not only on revenues but also indicators such as total number of hospitalized patients and proportion of big and medium operations, etc. When priorities were given to these evaluative indicators with dubious validity, who is there to care whether a patient has been given proper medical care before admission, whether wound pain needs to be relieved by medication after discharge, or whether follow-up visits be done on time?

The Chinese medical authorities have been attempting to establish a more reasonably graded medical system, allowing patients to get continuing medical services suitable for their diseases. However, the current system under construction does not help much in solving the above problems. The incompatibility of health information systems of various medical facilities alone is already a huge barrier to cross for medical institutions to network. In addition, each medical institution is an independent legal entity managed by different government departments, which further increases the difficulty of resource integration and collaboration.

Is this really an unsolvable problem, given the circumstances above mentioned? Surely not. China is now ranked second in the world in overall economic power. Not only does China have a large and powerful medical administration, but also an incredible social governance and control system. Why can't we learn from the various coordination mechanisms formed during the COVID-19 pandemic, which efficiently "locked down" cities with millions of people overnight, and carry out national-level design work to establish a truly effective graded medical system to solve the problem?

As the old saying goes, "rocks from other hills may serve to polish jade". In developed countries such as Japan, a medical system with public hospitals as the main body has long been established, and the Commonwealth countries represented by Canada and Australia also established a mature referral system between family doctors, local clinics, central hospitals, specialist physicians. China's medical authorities surely should and can draw lessons from experiences that these foreign counterparts have accumulated in medical system design through years of exploration and practice. China is now fully capable of establishing a graded medical system that's comparable to those in developed countries, which promise a solution to the discontinuity between inpatient services and pre-hospital and post-hospital medical services.

Regardless top-level design and implementation paths, to establish an effective graded medical system, the most critical is sufficient funding, especially for the local medical departments, so as to attract competent medical workers to devote themselves to primary medical services. One of the key reasons why the current graded medical system is not so successful is that local medical departments have been under funded, shaking the foundation of the grade medical system. On the other hand, hospitals, especially large and central ones, should also commit efforts to designing more humanized clinical pathways, and proactively connect pre-and post-hospital support for patients.

Another solution is to open the pre-hospital and post-hospital supporting business services to private institutions. The market demand is far from being met. Recently, a popular "consultation accompany" service, which means accompanying the patient to see a doctor, has emerged among the middle classes in Beijing and other big cities, a clear sign of the need for such services. If this new type of business can be gradually developed, an effective market-based solution to the above problems may be insight. Or, at least, it will provide a useful supplement to the graded medical system dominated by public medical care.

让医疗步入公众视野

主编导读（十六）

从量变到质变：国内临床研究40年发展之路

我曾经历过20世纪80～90年代国内的临床研究，那时候很少有拿得出手的临床论文，投稿到国际性刊物时心里还是相当发怵。想不到国内的临床和科研发展如此之快，随着经济现状和医院设施的快速改善，曾经极为羡慕的仪器、设备和手术器械很快在国内医院里普及开来，各种手术实施例数也开始超过国外著名医院，我们很有幸地见证了这个时代。但是新的问题来了，我们大部分的临床研究还处于以量取胜的状态，搞病例数轰炸，动不动就来个数百例、上千例报道。这种现象刚开始还真是"镇住"了国外杂志和专家，认为这是个"大数据"；但久而久之，我们文章的内在质量和学术上的不足等缺陷就暴露出来。而我们再看西方国家，哪怕是日本的文章，例数虽然不如我们多，但文章的质量和学术水平常常做得非常高、有声有色。在操作技术上，我们的文章还在津津乐道于手术技巧的展示，而发达国家可能更加注重的是理念的宣讲。不可否认，我们的临床科研文章已经有了很大的进步，但如何更进一步完成从以量取胜到质、量兼备的进化？这是一个必须重视、应该认真讨论的问题。

*HBSN*杂志本次请到北京大学肿瘤医院的著名外科教授邢宝才主任，他在这个方面有自己独到的思考和见解，写下本文与我们临床医生们进行分享。

从量变到质变：
国内临床研究报道的必经之路

徐　达　　邢宝才

北京大学肿瘤医院暨北京市肿瘤防治研究所肝胆胰外一科
恶性肿瘤发病机制及转化研究教育部重点实验室

经过近40年的改革开放，我国的医学发展突飞猛进，在大多数的医学领域，国内的诊治手段已经能够比肩国际，这种成就是有目共睹的。

近些年来随着医学研究队伍不断扩大，实验室研究设备及方法更加先进，我们取得了一些有影响力的研究成果并获得了国际的公认，但是整体来看，国内的高水平医学原创研究，特别是拥有高级别循证医学证据的临床研究仍落后于西方国家。我国人口基数大，多种疾病的发病人数在世界范围位居前列，若能充分利用这些患者资源，是非常便于开展疾病发病机制和诊断治疗相关研究的。

但目前一些临床报道仍处于以量取胜的状态，文章内在质量不高，无法取得足以改变临床实践的研究成果。那么，我国的临床研究如何加快从量变到质变的过程？下面我们将从四个方面对这一问题进行探讨。

临床科研人才的培养

由于我国人口基数大，临床医生人数众多，临床医生的科研能力存在参差不齐的现象，导致我们有一些没有接受过规范临床科研培训的医生人群，他们不具备进行临床研究的能力。要改变这种现状，我们首先要在临床医学教育过程中加强对于年轻临床医生的科研思维、科研方法以及科研意识的培养。

临床科研人员的科研素养和能力是解决临床问题的需要，是临床医学发展的原动力，这些培养包括文献检索与阅读、研究选题与设计、实验方法以及数据分析等。

具备了这些能力，临床医生才能有意识地发现问题，并针对临床问题设计规范的临床研究方案。

同时，要想改变临床研究文章数量多但质量不高的现象，我们需要改变单纯地将发表文章的数量与临床医生的职业发展相关联的局面。

当临床医生在工作中发现与临床相关的关键问题需要通过科研来解决时，我们可以组织建立研究团队，团队中拥有研究经验的医生和科研人员有针对性地进行科研课题设计和组织实施，使年轻的临床医生获取研究经验而保持对临床科研的敏锐性。另外，通过开办临床研究科研课题申报相关的培训课程，使临床医生顺利申请到资助；对于医院优势学科以及有前沿创新想法的人才，如果能给予政策上及启动经费上的支持，会帮助他们顺利地进行临床研究。

临床科研创新性的提高

目前我国临床研究每年发表的文章数量在世界范围内位于前列，但我们应该避免盲目跟风、单纯重复，提高原创性和创新性。

当我们临床医生具备了良好科研素质以及科研意识后，应该善于利用广泛的病例资源，发挥自己临床经验丰富的优势，在日常工作中发现新颖且有临床研究意义的问题，把着眼点放在如何解决临床问题上。

外科医生应该勇于承担，对于发现的科学问题，应该广泛阅读文献，结合研究进展，积极探索新技术、新方法，设计严谨的前瞻性或者回顾性多中心研究进行验证，得到高级别的循证医学证据，进而改写指南与共识。

在临床研究工作中应该积极"引进来，走出去"，建设科研交流平台，积极与国内及国际高水平中心学习交流、开阔视野，了解国

守在生命的边缘
医者沉思录

内外研究前沿及进展，使研究内容与国际上的热点难点接轨。

此外，对于临床问题，应该透过现象看本质，以临床为基础，构建科研与临床相结合的思路，积极与基础研究人员合作，进行机制探索，更好地阐述疾病的发生和发展过程。

临床科研平台的搭建

目前，虽然我国很多的临床研究中纳入病例数较多，但有时由于临床资料信息不全，使得研究结论比较浅显，形成不了改进指南的高级别证据。其原因与没有建立完善的临床数据库有关。

一个完整的临床科研平台以及数据库的搭建，是一个长期且艰难的积累过程，但这也是医学研究由简单重复到高水平研究的必经之路。这个过程需要团队成员具有良好的团队精神，进行长期的积累，具备长远规划的眼光，进行前瞻性的设计。当然，良好科研平台还需要病理、放射、超声等多学科的通力协作，才能最大限度地保证科研数据库的完整性和规范性。所以，科学研究需要踏实认真的数据积累，才能呈现高水平的研究成果。目前已经有很多中国学者在临床数据库建设以及高水平研究设计方面作出了很好的榜样。

东方肝胆外科医院程树群教授曾联合国内多中心，共同开展的一项关于合并门脉癌栓的可切除肝细胞肝癌（hepatocellular carcinoma，HCC）患者进行术前放疗的RCT（randomized controlled trial，随机对照试验）研究，研究结果发表于 *Journal of Clinical Oncology* 杂志。中山大学附属肿瘤医院的石明教授报道了其对所在中心合并门脉侵犯的HCC患者进行肝动脉灌注联合索拉非尼治疗对比单纯索拉非尼治疗的一项RCT研究，结果发表于 *JAMA Oncology* 杂志。

这些高水平研究都因其严谨的设计、翔实的分析和可靠的结果得到了国内国际同行的广泛认可和好评，并有可能改写指南，值得我们学习借鉴。

临床科研的使命感

尽管近年来我国医学发展已经达到较高水平，但临床上还存在很多悬而未决的问题。临床医生应该有一种使命感，这种使命感除了应该尽己所能地为患者解除病痛，也应该积极探索目前临床诊治过程中存在的问题，并想办法分析和解决问题。

正如希波克拉底誓言中所说的：我将分享我的医学知识，造福患者和推动医学进步。

进行临床研究的目的不仅是发表高水平的文章，更主要的是应该基于临床、服务临床、解决临床中的实际问题。任何一项临床研究成果的目的都应该是使患者得到更规范的治疗，从而使治疗获益最大化。这种使命感有助于临床医生的心态从被动研究到主动探索问题的方向转变。只有这样才能取得更多创新的、高水平的、真正解决临床问题的研究成果。目前我国的部分临床医学研究正如 Goh 和 Farrell 所分析，已经逐渐从以量取胜的状态得到改善。但是长期以来，临床指南的制定以及学科发展方向主要由西方研究学者主导。

虽然我国是非英文母语国家，我国学者要在高水平英文杂志上发表其研究成果，并得到国际研究领域的认可，语言上存在劣势。但在这种情况下，我国近年来的医学研究水平还是有了巨大的提高，发表了很多研究论文；并且从科研创新以及科研成果转化方面，形成了很好的科研氛围。

尽管目前仍存在一些问题，但是前期的积累是我们未来发展的基础，临床科研发展从量到质的转变，是一个长期、但是必须经历的过程。随着我们认识的提高，希望我国的临床研究逐步朝着拥有更高质量、创新性强并解决患者实际问题的方向发展。

参考文献

[1] Gao R, Liao Z, Li ZS. Scientific publications in gastroenterology and hepatology journals from Chinese authors in various parts of North Asia: 10-year survey of

literature. J Gastroenterol Hepatol 2008;23:374-8.

［2］Ba DN. We should pay more attention on clinical research. Zhonghua Yi Xue Za Zhi 2003; 83: 1-2.

［3］Wei X, Jiang Y, Zhang X, et al. Neoadjuvant Three-Dimensional Conformal Radiotherapy for Resectable Hepatocellular Carcinoma With Portal Vein Tumor Thrombus: A Randomized, Open-Label, Multicenter Controlled Study. J Clin Oncol 2019; 37: 2141-51.

［4］He M, Li Q, Zou R, et al. Sorafenib Plus Hepatic Arterial Infusion of Oxaliplatin, Fluorouracil, and Leucovorin vs Sorafenib Alone for Hepatocellular Carcinoma With Portal Vein Invasion: A Randomized Clinical Trial. JAMA Oncol 2019; 5: 953-60.

［5］Markel H. "I swear by Apollo" -on taking the Hippocratic oath. N Engl J Med 2004; 350: 2026-9.

［6］Goh KL, Farrell GC. Publications from China: the sleeping giant awakens. J Gastroenterol Hepatol 2008; 23: 341-3.

Quality over quantity: a necessary path for clinical research transformation in China

Xu Da, Xing Baocai

Key Laboratory of Carcinogenesis and Translational Research (Ministry of Education/Beijing), Hepatopancreatobiliary Surgery Department I, Peking University Cancer Hospital & Institute, Beijing, China

Since the Chinese economic reform in 1978, its medical field has made remarkable progress in the past 40 years. In most medical fields, China's diagnosis and treatment methods are comparable to the international high standards. In recent years, with the continuous expansion of the medical research team and the improvement of laboratory research equipment and methods, China has achieved some influential and internationally recognized research outcomes. However, overall, China still lags behind developed countries in terms of high-level original medical research, especially in high evidence-based medical research [1].

China has a large population base, and the number of cases is among the highest in the world. If Chinese doctors can make full use of these patient resources, it would be very beneficial to conduct research on disease pathogenesis and diagnosis and treatment. However, many clinical studies currently focus on quantity rather than quality, so it is difficult to obtain research results that can change clinical practice. There are subjective and objective factors leading to this situation. What is the future of clinical research in China? This question will be discussed from the following four aspects.

Clinical research training for young clinicians

A big issue with Chinese clinicians is that many of them have not received standardized clinical research training and they lack the basic skills to conduct clinical research. To change this situation, it is necessary to emphasize the importance of cultivating scientific research thinking, methods, and awareness in young clinicians in the process of clinical medical education. Clinicians need to improve their clinical research literacy because it helps to solve clinical problems and it prompts the development of modern medicine. Only when clinicians have scientific research capabilities such as literature retrieval and reading, topic selection and research design, data analysis, and maintaining enthusiasm as well as sensitivity to scientific research in clinical work, can clinicians consciously discover problems in their work and design standardized research for clinical problems. Besides, in China, the number of articles is often associated with the professional development of clinicians in most of the medical institutions, which leads clinicians to publish as many articles as possible, regardless of the quality of the articles. The management department of medical scientific research ought to reinforce their communication with front-line clinicians, devoting more efforts on improving the scientific research ability of clinical researchers. They could also provide financial supports and preferential policy based on the needs of clinicians, solve the problems encountered by clinical researchers in their research, and proactively held more clinical research training courses related to the clinical scientific research project application. For those who have innovative ideas and some advantageous departments, the hospital can also give them more support to help conducting high-level clinical research smoothly.

Innovations in clinical research

A large number of clinical studies are published in China every year, but many studies are still blindly following the trend, simply repetitive, and lack originality and innovation. After having good scientific research training and awareness, Chinese clinicians could make good use of our large patient resources, taking advantage of our valuable clinical experience, and exploring novel and significant clinical research problems in our daily work. The most important thing is to focus on how to solve clinical problems. Clinicians should have the courage to discover scientific problems in the clinic, read the literature extensively, actively explore new technologies and methods based on the research progress, design rigorous prospective or retrospective multi-center studies for verification, obtain high-level evidence-based medicine, and eventually rewrite the guidelines and consensus. In daily work, we could actively "bring in and go out", building scientific research communicate platform, actively communicating with domestic and international high-level centers, broadening our horizons and understanding the frontiers of domestic and foreign research, so that we can integrate our research with the international hotspots. In addition, for clinical problems, clinicians need to see through the appearance to perceive the essence, combining scientific research with clinical practice. We can actively cooperate with basic medical researchers to explore mechanisms to better explain the occurrence and progression of diseases [2].

Establishment of the clinical research platform

At present, many Chinese clinical studies have included a large number of cases, but their clinical information is not comprehensive. Some of the research conclusions drawn are relatively simple, which cannot form high-level evidence to change the guidelines. The reason is due to the lack of a thorough clinical database. Establishing an integrated clinical research platform and database is a long and difficult accumulation process, but it is the only way for clinical research to go from simple repetition to high-level research. This integrating process requires a group of people with good team spirit, long-term data accumulation, and a long-term vision for designing leading medical research. Of course, a good research platform also requires the concerted efforts of pathology, radiology, ultrasound and other disciplines to work together to ensure the integrity and standardization of the research database to the greatest extent. Therefore, scientific research requires solid data accumulation in order to gain high-level research results. Up to now, many Chinese clinicians have made good examples in the development of clinical database and performing high-level scientific research. Wei et al. published a randomized controlled trial (RCT) on preoperative radiotherapy for resectable hepatocellular carcinoma (HCC) with portal vein tumor thrombus based on their database of HCC, combining with several other centers [3]. He et al. reported the results of their center, by conducting an RCT study of hepatic arterial infusion combined with sorafenib versus sorafenib alone for the treatment of HCC patients with portal vein invasion [4]. These high-quality researches have been recognized and praised by international peers for the rigorous design, detailed data analysis and solid results of the study, which is possible to rewrite the guidelines.

Obligation in clinical research

In China, although medical development has reached a high level in recent years, it is still far from meeting people's needs, and there are still many unresolved problems in clinical practice. Clinicians should have a sense of obligation, not only do their best to relieve the pain of patients but also actively identify and try to find ways to solve the existing problems in current clinical diagnosis and treatment process. Just as we said in the

Hippocratic Oath, *"as long as my life endures, may I commit myself to advance the nation's medical science and research as well as the well-being of the entire human race"* [5].

Publishing high-level articles is not the only purpose of conducting clinical research. More importantly, we hope the research could solve practical problems in the clinic, so that more patients can receive more beneficial standardized treatment. With this sense of obligation in clinical research, clinicians can change their mindset from passively conducting research to actively exploring problems, and only then can they obtain more innovative, high-level research outcomes that truly solve clinical problems.

For a long time, the development of clinical medical research in China has been mainly focused on quantity of the research [6]. However, we should admit that western clinicians have long been playing main role in evidence-based clinical guideline making. It is quite difficult for Chinese scholars, which are non-native English speakers to report their results and publish research in high-level journals to gain wide recognition from Western countries. Indeed, clinical research in China has made great progress in recent years. We have also gradually overcome the difficulties in hardware and caught up in the amount of research. The government and scientific research institutions also made great efforts to encourage scientific research innovation and the output of scientific research results, which had formed a superior scientific research atmosphere. Many of the importance research results has been recognized and accepted by worldwide academic community. The prior experiences set the foundation for the discovery of new findings in future development. Transformation of clinical research from quantity to quality is a long and necessary process. With the improvement of our understanding, future clinical research will definitely move towards high-quality, innovative research and solve the real problems for patients in China.

References

［1］Gao R, Liao Z, Li ZS. Scientific publications in gastroenterology and hepatology journals from Chinese authors in various parts of North Asia: 10-year survey of literature. J Gastroenterol Hepatol 2008; 23: 374-8.

［2］Ba DN. We should pay more attention on clinical research. Zhonghua Yi Xue Za Zhi 2003; 83: 1-2.

［3］Wei X, Jiang Y, Zhang X, et al. Neoadjuvant Three-Dimensional Conformal Radiotherapy for Resectable Hepatocellular Carcinoma With Portal Vein Tumor Thrombus: A Randomized, Open-Label, Multicenter Controlled Study. J Clin Oncol 2019; 37: 2141-51.

［4］He M, Li Q, Zou R, et al. Sorafenib Plus Hepatic Arterial Infusion of Oxaliplatin, Fluorouracil, and Leucovorin vs Sorafenib Alone for Hepatocellular Carcinoma With Portal Vein Invasion: A Randomized Clinical Trial. JAMA Oncol 2019; 5: 953-60.

［5］Markel H. "I swear by Apollo" -on taking the Hippocratic oath. N Engl J Med 2004; 350: 2026-9.

［6］Goh KL, Farrell GC. Publications from China: the sleeping giant awakens. J Gastroenterol Hepatol 2008; 23: 341-3.

主编导读（十七）

每天都说的DRG到底是什么？该怎么用？你想知道的都在这里了

我第一次听到DRG这一词汇时浑然不知这代表了什么意思，那是数年前被卫生部的一个下属机构请去做疾病和手术名称分类时才了解到的，我和其他两位外科医生负责肝胆胰疾病方面的内容，当时是为了中国开展DRG工作做准备。

后来才慢慢清楚，DRG是Diagnosis Related Groups的缩写，即按疾病诊断相关分组，这个名词看起来只是一个疾病分类方面的概念，但是实际上和规范目前的医疗收费系统有很大的关系。通俗一点讲，就是按照疾病的分类和治疗对病种的总体费用进行打包，如肝癌要进行右半肝切除，DRG会给出一个治疗总体费用的指导价（如多少万元），如果医院在治疗过程中费用大大超出DRG所规范的指标，那么医院就有可能要支付多出来的费用；反之，如果治疗肝癌行右半肝切除，总体所花的费用低于DRG的指导价（一般指导价会定得宽松一点），医保系统就会返回多出的钱给医院作为奖励。理论上这么做，对于阻止医疗乱收费用、鼓励减少不必要的消耗、奖励做得好的医务人员是有帮助的，并且也间接地鼓励减少并发症的发生（有并发症住院时间、治疗费用都会增高）、缩短患者的住院时间等。

实际上这种DRG定价、收费模式不是什么新的概念，在发达国家一直在开展，而且经过不断地改良和修正变得更加成熟和完善。在我们国家已经有了初步的试用版，并且正在国内的一些医院里进行试运行。当时无法确认的是这个听起来相对有道理，又在其他国家运行了多年的收费系统能不能在我国顺利开展，是不是会有水土不服的情况产生。

当我和同事们聊起这个中国的DRG时，惊讶地发现身边的各级外科医生们还都不知道这个正在国内慢慢展开的DRG项目，我萌发了一个想法，就是应该向世界和国内介绍我国的DRG开展情况。为此，我专门拜访了我国负责DRG项目的专家于丽华主任，请她执笔为我们概要介绍中国的DRG的特点和开展的现状。

按DRG定价支付医疗费用：
我们走到哪一步了？

于丽华　　郎婧婧

国家卫生健康委卫生发展研究中心　医药成本价格研究部

按疾病诊断相关分组（Diagnosis Related Groups，DRG）是目前国际上比较公认的一种先进的现代化管理方法，20世纪60年代末由耶鲁大学首创，1983年被美国Medicare用于住院预付费体系中，之后被澳大利亚、德国、法国、英国、日本、韩国、北欧等发达国家引入之后一些东欧、亚非拉的发展中国家也相继引入，广泛应用于定价支付、预算管理、绩效评价与比较等领域。

DRG作为一种精细化管理工具，结合相应的付费机制，可以有效满足医疗费用控制、医院管理和医保管理的要求，对推进支付方式从后付制转向预付制、促进医疗系统改善绩效管理具有重要意义。

DRG概念及应用领域

DRG是按照疾病严重程度、治疗方法的复杂程度以及资源消耗程度的相似性，将住院患者分成一定数量的疾病组，以实现不同的管理目标。

DRG原则上要覆盖所有的住院患者（除罕见病、精神、中医、创新技术等特殊情况），决定患者分到哪一个组的最主要因素是患者本次住院的主要诊断和采取的主要治疗方式（手术操作），以及其他如患者是否有合并症/并发症、住院天数、年龄等要素，综合这些因素，资源消耗相似的患者可以分在一个组内，住院疾病一般可以被分为600 ～ 2000个疾病组。

一个国家或一个地区可以对本地区医疗机构，以已经确定好的

DRG组为单位，进行收付费管理或医保支付管理、绩效考核以及对该地区所有医疗机构资金进行分配与管理等。

中国DRG版本介绍

2017年我国开始试点，目前国家层面主要有以下三种用途。

（1）用于收付费管理的C-DRG

共包含900个DRG组，其特点如下。

1）由中国的临床医生结合中国疾病谱特征，按临床相似性进行分组，以国家卫生健康委财务司《全国医疗服务成本与价格监测与研究网络》中1400余家医疗机构的费用和成本数据进行验证，确定最终分组。

2）创新规范了供临床医生使用的《中国临床疾病诊断规范术语集》（CCDT）和《中国医疗服务操作分类与编码》（CCHI）作为分组的标准工具，并将上述工具和ICD-10疾病分类、ICD-9-CM-3手术操作分类进行对接，便于医院管理。

3）在全国首创按DRG收费和付费一体化改革，即每个DRG组均对应一个价格，医院提供服务后按DRG组的价格收费，医保按DRG组的价格制定医保支付比例进行支付。

（2）用于医保付费管理的CHS-DRG

国家医保局于2019年在全国30个试点城市推行的DRG付费改革，使用CHS-DRG版本，该版DRG共包含376个核心DRG组（A-DRG），618个细分DRG组，使用医保版ICD-10和ICD-9-CM-3作为分组工具。

（3）用于绩效评价管理的CN-DRG

国家卫生健康委医政医管局在2013年推行的应用DRG开展医院绩效评价，使用CN-DRG版本，共包含804个DRG组，使用国家临床版2.0 ICD-10和ICD-9-CM-3作为分组工具。在2019年启动的三级公立医院绩效考核中也引入CN-DRG进行指标设计和评价。

DRG收付费改革的实践与应用

我国长期以来实行的是按项目收付费的制度，即以医疗服务项目为计价单位，医院根据向患者提供的服务进行累加收费，其特点是医院收入与提供的服务量直接相关，与疾病诊疗的主要诊断和主要操作无关，缺点是容易诱导患者消费。

按DRG收付费是以分好的疾病组为单位，预先制定每个组的价格用于医院收费和医保付费，该疾病组的价格包括了患者从入院到出院整个过程中开展的医疗服务及使用的药品和卫生材料，医保方按该价格和医保的支付比例向医院支付费用，医院方也按同样的价格和患者的自付比例向患者收费。而每一个患者进入哪个DRG组，或者说按哪个DRG组收付费，与这个患者出院最终确定的主要诊断和主要操作密切相关，而与他做了多少个项目无关。

DRG收付费改革方案的特点是每个DRG组的价格是事先确定好的，所有的药品、耗材均变成了医院的成本，其运行的基本原则是：超支不补，结余归己。这种政策的执行极大地促进了医院运营从注重扩大收入转向注重成本管控，激发医院规范行为、控制成本的内生动力，使医疗机构在保证患者质量安全的情况下，主动改变行为，控制成本，提高效率，以获得最大的结余。例如一位有合并症的原发性肝细胞癌患者住院期间主要进行了根治性肝癌肝叶切除术，按项目收费时，根据患者实施的服务项目进行累加，总费用在4万～10万元不等。实行DRG管理后该类患者被分入"肝脏的复杂手术，有合并症并发症"DRG组，以某试点地区为例其收付费标准统一为8万元，医院根据临床实际结合临床路径提供适宜的服务及药品耗材，只要进入这个组的患者一律按8万元结算。因此，医疗机构要大力提高医院精细化管理水平，规范医生诊疗行为，合理控制成本，促进医院和医务人员获得收益。

未来应用的展望

我国近几年持续深化医改，在支付方式改革方面的力度逐年加大，成效显著，结合国际DRG实施的经验以及我国现状，我国未来DRG改革的趋势如下。

（1）统一版本

从国家层面发布统一的DRG版本，以及统一的疾病分类和手术操作等分组工具，无论将DRG应用到哪个领域，从国家层面版本要保持一致，才能使用统一的信息语言进行比较和发展。

（2）监测体系

形成基于DRG上报数据的全国统一的监测体系，监督医疗服务行为规范、防范医保基金风险，也为开展院际和专科间的比较分析提供信息平台。

（3）调整机制

建立长期的动态调整机制，对DRG分组、分组工具、支付标准和配套政策进行定期的更新和调整。

（4）有针对性

未来的医保支付方式改革趋势是实行多元复合式的支付方式，没有一种支付方式能够包打天下，一定是针对不同医疗服务特点，推进不同的支付方式改革。

（5）明确主体

要坚持和明确，医务人员才是支付方式改革的主体，所有的支付方式改革都要遵循临床规律，尊重临床规范，统一医务人员的诊断和操作标准，由医务人员对诊疗信息负主体责任，才能有效规范和真实地反映诊疗行为，为未来实施收付费改革一体化奠定基础。

参考文献

［1］Fetter RB, Shin Y, Freeman JL, et al. Case mix definition by diagnosis-related groups. Med Care 1980; 18: iii, 1-53.

［2］Busse R, Geissler A, Quentin W, et al. Diagnosis-related groups in Europe: moving towards transparency, efficiency and quality in hospitals. Maidenhead: Open University Press, 2011: 3-41.

[3] Zhang ZZ, Jiang Q, Yu LH. The overall design for the pricing and payment regulation on Chinese Diagnosis Related Groups. Chinese Health Economics 2017; 36: 5-8.

[4] Langenbrunner JC, Cashin C, O'Dougherty S. Designing and implementing health care provider payment systems: how-to manual. Washington DC: The World Bank, 2009: 6-7.

Diagnosis-related Groups (DRG) pricing and payment policy in China: where are we?

Yu Lihua, Lang Jingjing

Healthcare Cost and Price Division, China National Health Development Research Center of National Health Commission, Beijing, China

Diagnosis-related Groups (DRG) is an internationally recognized advanced hospital management method. It was pioneered by Yale University in the late 1960s and has been used as the inpatient prospective payment system by the U.S. Medicare program since 1983 [1,2]. It has since been introduced in Australia, Germany, France, the UK, Japan, South Korea, and Scandinavia. It is widely used in the fields of pricing and payment, budget allocation, performance evaluation, and comparison [2]. As a refined hospital management tool, DRG combined with the corresponding payment mechanism can effectively meet the requirements of health expenditure control, hospital management, and health insurance management [3]. DRG is also crucial for promoting the shift of payment methods from retrospective payment to prospective payment and for improving the performance management of the healthcare system.

The DRG concept

DRG divides inpatients into a certain number of disease groups according to the severity of the diseases, the complexity of the treatment methods, and the homogeneity of the resource consumption to achieve a variety management goals [1,2]. In principle, DRG should cover all hospitalized patients, except for special patients with rare diseases, mental illness, or those treated with special regimens, such as Traditional Chinese Medicine, cutting-edge technology etc. The most important factors in determining which group a patient is assigned to is the principal diagnosis and principal procedure. Comorbidities and complications, length of stay, age, and other factors should also be considered. Hospitalization diseases can generally be divided into 600 to 2,000 disease groups [2]. A country or a region can use DRG as a tool to conduct pricing and payment management, budget allocation, hospital performance evaluation, and comparison.

Introduction of DRG versions to China

In China, Beijing initially took the lead in DRG research by piloting a program in 2003. Since then, Zhejiang Province, Yunnan Province, Shenyang Province, Shanghai Municipal Province, and other cities have developed their respective local DRG versions and have actively piloted programs in the fields of payment and hospital performance evaluation.

The Chinese government mandated the inception of DRG piloting at the national level in 2017. At present, there are three main versions at the national level. The first version implemented was the C-DRG, which is used for pricing and payment. In 2017, the National Health Commission launched the C-DRG, comprising a total of 900 DRG groups, to reform pricing and payment in the cities of Sanming, Shenzhen, and Karamay, and three piloting hospitals in Fujian Province [3]. The C-DRG has three primary characteristics. First, its DRG groups patients mainly according to clinical similarity, verified by the expenditure and cost data of more than 1,400 medical institutions reported in the "National Healthcare Cost and Price Monitoring and Research Network" which was established by the Finance Department of National Health Commission. Second, to facilitate hospital management, the C-DRG innovatively uses two DRG grouping tools, "Chinese Clinical Disease Terminology" (CCDT) and "Chinese Classification of Health Interventions" (CCHI) by mapping these tools to the International Classification of Disease (ICD)-10 and ICD-9-CM-3. Third, the C-DRG uses DRG groups as the unit to charge patients in all hospitals with a standard price, which is in turn paid via health insurance; this system represents the first successful reform of healthcare payment in China [3].

The second version of DRG which has been implemented in China is the CHS-DRG, which is used for health insurance payment. In 2019, the National Healthcare Security Administration launched the DRG payment reform in 30 piloting cities across the country, using the CHS-DRG which comprises a total of 376 adjacent-DRG groups and 618 DRG subgroups. The CHS-DRG uses the ICD-10 and ICD-9-CM-3 (National Healthcare Security Version) as its the grouping tools. The National Healthcare Security Administration proposed a DRG payment reform to conduct simulated piloting in 30 cities in 2020 and actual piloting in 2021.

The third version that has been employed in China is the CN-DRG, which is used for hospital performance evaluation and administration. In 2013, the Bureau of Medical Administration of National Health Commission launched the DRG on hospital performance evaluation, using the CN-DRG which comprises a total of 804 DRG groups and the ICD-10 and ICD-9-CM-3 (National Clinical Version 2.0) as grouping tools. The performance evaluation scope covers nearly 1,000 hospitals across 29 provinces and municipalities. In 2019, the CN-DRG was also introduced for indicator design in the performance examination of tertiary public hospitals.

DRG pricing and payment reform

For an extended period of time, healthcare payment in China has consisted of a fee-for-service payment method. In this system, the hospital is reimbursed by health insurance for each individual health care service provided and, to provide each service, the hospital is permitted to bill purchasers for all expenditures incurred [3,4]. The payment is directly related to the number of services, and thus the hospital is incentivized to increase the number of overall services during a patient's hospitalization [4].

The DRG pricing and payment reform uses the DRG group as the unit of pricing. With this system, the price of the service that hospitals bill purchasers is predetermined. The price of each group includes the healthcare services, drugs, and medical consumables provided from admission to discharge. The hospital is reimbursed by health insurance according to the DRG price and the reimbursement ratio. The hospital also bills the patient according to the same price and the out-of-pocket payment ratio. Which DRG group each patient is assigned to is closely related to the principal diagnosis and principal procedure during the hospitalization, and is not related to the number health care services received, or drugs or medical consumables used. The characteristic of DRG pricing and payment reform is that the price of each DRG group is determined in advance. All costs related to services, drugs, and consumables are to be borne by the hospital. The basic billing principle of DRG reform is that "excess expenditures will no longer be reimbursed and the balance will be retained". Therefore, the reform will emphatically promote the transformation of the Chinese hospital operation model from a focus on expanding revenue to a focus on cost control and optimization. It will also motivate hospitals to standardize diagnosis and treatment, improve efficiency, and ensure quality and safety.

An example is perhaps useful to illustrate the reformed process and its intended effects: a group of patients are diagnosed with primary hepatocellular carcinoma with comorbidities and undergo radical lobectomy as treatment during the hospitalization. Under the fee-for-

守在生命的边缘
医者沉思录

service payment system, the expenditures for hospitalization range between 40,000 and 100,000 CNY for different patients according to the healthcare services, drugs, and medical consumables provided. Under the reformed DRG pricing and payment system, these patients would be classified into the DRG group named "major liver procedures with comorbidities and complications". Taking a piloting city as an example, the price of this DRG group would 80,000 CNY, and patients assigned to this DRG group would be billed at 80,000 CNY regardless of the services, drugs, and consumables received. In providing these to the patient, the hospital would need to greatly refine their management of resources, standardize clinicians' diagnosis and treatment, and control costs to ensure quality while keeping expenditures low.

Prospects for future applications

China has intensified the degree of reform to its healthcare system in recent years, with the efforts to transform healthcare payment increasing each year and yielding remarkable success. According to the international experiences of DRG application and the current healthcare status of China, the future measures of DRG reform should include the following: first, a unified DRG grouping regulation and unified grouping tools for disease and health intervention classification on the national level should be published. Regardless to which field the DRG is applied, the version should be sufficiently consistent to facilitate comparisons between hospitals using standard terms and criteria. Second, a nationally unified monitoring system based on minimal DRG data should be established to monitor the diagnosis and treatment behaviors. This would aid in minimizing the risks of health insurance funding, and provide an information platform for conducting interhospital and interspecialty comparative analysis. Third, a long-term dynamic mechanism should be developed to regularly update DRG grouping, grouping tools, payment standards, and supporting policies. Fourth, multiple payment methods based on the characteristics of different healthcare services should be supported. Finally, it should be emphasized that clinicians are the linchpin in the revolution of healthcare payment. As all payment methods need to follow clinical norms, the classifications and terminologies of diagnosis and procedures should be unified at the national level. It is the responsibility of clinicians to effectively standardize and adopt sound diagnosis and treatment practices, as these form the foundation on which the future pricing and payment standards will be built.

References

[1] Fetter RB, Shin Y, Freeman JL, et al. Case mix definition by diagnosis-related groups. Med Care 1980; 18: iii, 1-53.

[2] Busse R, Geissler A, Quentin W, et al. Diagnosis-related groups in Europe: moving towards transparency, efficiency and quality in hospitals. Maidenhead: Open University Press, 2011: 3-41.

[3] Zhang ZZ, Jiang Q, Yu LH. The overall design for the pricing and payment regulation on Chinese Diagnosis Related Groups. Chinese Health Economics 2017; 36: 5-8.

[4] Langenbrunner JC, Cashin C, O'Dougherty S. Designing and implementing health care provider payment systems: how-to manual. Washington DC: The World Bank, 2009: 6-7.

主编导读（十八）

中国的医疗保障：什么秘诀照顾了14亿人民？

即使我在医疗领域里工作了那么多年，对于我国的医保体系仍一直处于不甚知晓和理解的状态。可能对于相当一部分民众和医务工作者也会体会到我们国家的医保系统是一个谜之存在。

我能感受到这些年来，医保经过了很大的改革，可能有了不少的进步，同时也听到不少人对于我们医保体系有着抱怨和不满。到底我们国家的医保体系是如何运作的，在世界上又归入哪个"流派"或者独门独派？其内幕又是怎样的？这些问题一直搁在心里的一个角落，没有动力、时间和精力去试图弄清楚。

直到这次新冠疫情暴发，我们惊讶地发现，实际上我们的基本医疗保障还是相当轧硬的。虽然有些人一定会有不同的看法，但是不可否认的事实是，对于突发而来的新冠疫情，这个保障系统在经过最初期的仓促和紊乱之后，就有能力把疫情控制得有声有色。反观我们一直崇拜的欧美医疗卫生系统，那些完善到没有进步空间的卫生保障系统却在一时间垮塌了，就像心中的灯塔垮塌。难道我们的医疗保障投入了更多的钱吗？

我查阅了世界卫生组织（WHO）发布的公开资料，惊讶地发现，美国的医疗卫生支出占到国内生产总值的17.06%之多，人均达到9403美元；而中国卫生支出仅占国内生产总值的5.15%，人均420美元，连世界平均水平的9.90%都不到。

这样的支出水平，想象中应该保证不了全国人民的基本健康需求，更加不用说来应对卫生系统的突发紧急事件。但是再看，我们国家的医疗保障系统虽然远不是完美的，存在不少缺陷和遗漏，但是总体上还是保障了全国14亿人民的基本医疗需求，尤其是在这次突发疫情面前显得如此稳健和有力，相比花了这么多钱还没有办好医疗的美国，我们难道有什么秘诀吗？

是因为医疗资源相对廉价？老百姓听话，还是实际上贴了很多钱？是我们的组织协调能力更胜一筹？或者是我们用钱浪费少，都花在刀口上？也许国家有其他的补贴没有被算进去？还是有人会说这种所谓的高效医保体系就是一个错觉。

为了寻求答案，给我们的读者一个比较标准的解释，我们就这些问题专门邀请了国家医疗保障局的专家，为我们解读中国的医疗保障制度的概况和发展，使我们医务工作者和广大民众有一个了解我国医保内幕的窗口。

中国的医疗保障：
什么秘诀照顾了14亿人民？

伊保康

中国国家医疗保障局　新闻办公室

医疗保障是减轻群众就医负担、增进民生福祉、维护社会和谐稳定的重大制度安排。我们建立全民医保制度的根本目的，就是要解除全体人民的疾病医疗后顾之忧。我们国家承担着世界上规模最大的基本医疗保障网，为全方位全周期维护人民群众健康作出了重要贡献。

中国医疗保障的构成、覆盖及运行态势

目前，我国医疗保障体系是一个以基本医疗保险为主体，医疗救助为托底，补充医疗保险、商业健康保险、慈善捐赠、医疗互助共同发展的多层次医疗保障体系。其中，基本医疗保险由两部分组成。包括职工医疗保险和城乡居民医疗保险。就业人员参加职工医疗保险，医保费由单位缴费和职工个人缴费两部分组成。非就业人员参加城乡居民医疗保险，医保费由政府补助和个人缴费共同组成。

2018年国家医保局成立后，持续完善全民医保体系，全面实现城乡居民医保统筹。截至2020年9月，基本医疗保险参保人数已经超过了13.5亿人，参保率稳定在95%以上，建成了世界上最大的医疗保障网。医保基金运行平稳，基金规模进一步扩大。2019年，全国基本医保基金（含生育保险）收入2.44万亿元，支出2.09万亿元。

医疗救助通过资助困难群众参加基本医疗保险，并对政策范围内个人、家庭难以承担的医疗费用给予补助等方式，确保困难群众公平获得基本医疗服务。自2018年以来，累计惠及贫困人口4.8亿人

次，帮助减轻其医疗负担金额近3300亿元，助力1000万因病致贫群众精准脱贫，实现贫困人口的基本医疗有保障。

此外，各类社会力量积极参与补充医疗保障，主要发挥市场机制的作用，成为多层次医疗保障体系的重要组成部分。

中国医疗保障体系的特色和优势

中国政府始终把人民身体健康和生命安全作为政府的基本职责，把基本医保作为公共产品向全民提供。尽管我国医疗保障筹资总额占GDP比重约2.5%的水平，与其他社会保险体制发达国家相比还有差距，但这个比例与人均GDP 1万美元的发展阶段总体是相适应的。

坚持尽力而为

首先是加大财政资金投入力度，2007－2019年国家财政将医疗保障支出从913亿元提高到8000亿元，当年财政支出占比从1.87%增长至3.50%。2020年居民医保人均财政补助标准达到550元。

其次是聚焦重点。聚焦对贫困人口实现基本医疗有保障的目标，持续加大资金投入力度，向贫困地区、贫困人口倾斜。建档立卡贫困人口参保率达到99.9%以上，经基本医保、大病保险、医疗救助三重制度综合保障后，贫困人口住院费用实际报销比例稳定在80%左右。

做到量力而行

不超过经济发展水平，不作过高承诺，既满足人民群众的基本需要，又避免福利化倾向，确保基金可持续运行。基本医疗保险不越位，也为补充医疗保险、商业健康保险等发展留足空间。

全力强化管理

多措并举。通过一系列"组合拳"管好人民群众"救命钱"，推动医保事业高质量发展。

强招采。基本形成常态化的国家组织药品集中采购和使用机制，三批药品国家集采共112个品种，平均降幅为54%，每年节约医药费用达539亿元。

启动国家组织高值医用耗材集中带量采购改革，连续4年完善医保药品目录，初步形成医保药品目录动态调整机制。将部分"僵尸药"调出目录，为更多临床价值高的药品进入目录腾出空间。

管支付。稳步推进医保支付方式改革，全国97.5%的统筹地区开展了医保总额控制，30个城市开展了DRG付费国家试点。

严监管。坚持重拳出击，两年共查处违规机构33万家次，追回资金125.6亿元；发挥飞行检查利器作用，2019年共派出69个飞行检查组赴全国30个省份开展实地检查，查出涉嫌违规资金22.32亿元；健全严密有力的基金监管机制，深入开展专项治理。

改善药品价格形成机制

国家医保局成立后，我们对医保药品目录实施了动态调整，并建立了调整规则，出台了《基本医疗保险用药管理暂行办法》。

我们坚持"保基本"的功能定位，用药保障水平与基本医疗保险基金和参保人承受能力相适应。对医保药品实现科学、规范、精细、动态管理。对于独家药品通过准入谈判的方式确定支付标准，不仅节约了医保资金，还显著降低了患者的费用负担。动态调整机制的建立，将便利更多好药及时纳入医保目录。

以治疗肝炎的药物为例，近年来，在有关部门的不懈努力下，病毒性肝炎治疗药物价格大幅降低。在2015年时，乙肝类抗病毒药物替诺福韦酯与恩替卡韦年人均治疗费用分别高达约20 000元和9000元。2018年，开展"4＋7"试点后，替诺福韦酯和恩替卡韦年人均治疗费用均降低至210 ～ 240元。

2019年开展试点扩围后，两种药品的年人均治疗费用进一步降低至70元左右。同年，国家医保局还对多种治疗丙肝的口服药物进行谈判并纳入医保报销范围。与谈判前相比，患者负担降低95%以上。

随着药品价格的大幅下降，慢性肝炎的诊断率和治疗率低的现状也得到了彻底改善。恩替卡韦集采后，"4＋7"试点城市的实际采购量超过上年度的3.5倍。

集采不仅使长期服药的患者负担减轻，而且让以往有病吃不起药的群众受益，显著提高了患者治疗的可及性，有助于实现世界卫生组织提出的"2030年消除病毒性肝炎对公共卫生的威胁"的目标。

建立健全多层次医疗保障体系

近年来，我国商业健康险以年30%的增速迅速发展。2019年商业健康保险原保费收入为7066亿元，同比增长29.7%。同时，各类补充医疗保障、慈善医疗救助快速发展。近年来蔚然兴起的医疗互助也为提升群众医疗保障水平贡献新生力量。

为适应新时代群众不断提高的健康需求，《中共中央国务院关于深化医疗保障制度改革的意见》提出，要强化基本医疗保险、大病保险与医疗救助三重保障功能，促进各类医疗保障互补衔接，提高重特大疾病和多元医疗需求保障水平。完善和规范居民大病保险、职工大额医疗费用补助、公务员医疗补助及企业补充医疗保险。加快发展商业健康保险，丰富健康保险产品供给，用足用好商业健康保险个人所得税政策，研究扩大保险产品范围。加强市场行为监管，突出健康保险产品设计、销售、赔付等关键环节监管，提高健康保障服务能力。

促进医疗保障高质量发展

今年是"十三五"收官之年，也是谋划"十四五"规划的关键之年。站在全面建成小康社会，开启建设社会主义现代化强国新征程的历史交汇点，我们需要对医疗保障面临的趋势和挑战有更加清醒的认识。

从人口年龄结构看，60岁以上老年人将在"十四五"末期超过3亿人，在职职工与退休人员的比例将持续下降，对医保基金的稳健运行提出严峻挑战。

从疾病风险看，在传染性疾病与慢性病双重负担下，基金支出压力持续存在。随着人民群众生活水平不断提高，对健康的需求也日益提高，医疗保障服务能力与广大人民群众的期盼还有一定差距。

医疗保障关系广大人民群众切身利益。"十四五"时期，我们将继续加强管理，优化服务，深化改革，不断创新，推动多层次医疗保障更加完善，引导医保、医疗、医药协同发展，促进医保制度更加成熟定型，让人民有更可靠、清晰的医保预期，增强人民群众的获得感、幸福感、安全感。

参考文献

［1］National Healthcare Security Development Report 2019. Available online: http://www.nhsa.gov.cn/art/2020/6/24/art_7_3268.html.

［2］What it means that the GDP per capita exceeds 10,000 US dollars. 2020. Available online: https://baijiahao.baidu.com/s?id=1656049179746010782&wfr=spider&for=pc.

［3］The Notice of Preparing Relevant Work of 2020 Residents Basic Medical Security, National Healthcare Security Administration, Ministry of Finance, State Taxation Administration. 2020. Available online: http://www.gov.cn/zhengce/zhengceku/2020-06/19/content_5520571.htm

［4］The "three-year action" of medical insurance poverty alleviation has reduced the burden of the poor by nearly 300 billion Yuan. 2020. Available online: http://www.xinhuanet.com/politics/2020-10/14/c_1126611738.htm.

［5］The state has made remarkable achievements in the centralized purchase of drugs, saving 53.9 billion yuan annually, and the average price of the purchased three batches of drugs has reduced more than half. 2020. Available online: http://sh.people.com.cn/n2/2020/1014/c138654-34348282.html.

［6］Interim measures for drug administration of basic medical insurance. 2020. Available online: http://www.gov.cn/zhengce/zhengceku/2020-08/04/content_5532409.htm.

［7］Data from China Banking and Insurance Regulatory Commission. Available online: http://www.cbirc.gov.cn/cn/view/pages/index/index.html.

［8］ Opinions on Deepening the Reform of Medical Security System, The CPC Central Committee, The State Council. 2020. Available online: http://www.gov.cn/zhengce/2020-03/05/content_5487407.htm.

［9］ Zheng Bingwen: China's elderly population will exceed 300 million at the end of the 14th Five-Year Plan. 2020. Available online: http://bgimg.ce.cn/xwzx/gnsz/gdxw/202010/27/t20201027_35939625.shtml.

An overview of the Chinese healthcare system

Yi Baokang

National Healthcare Security Administration, Beijing, China

The healthcare security system is an important institutional arrangement for reducing people's medical burden, improving people's well-being, and therefore maintaining social harmony and stability in China. The purpose of establishing a national medical security system is to relieve all people of their worries concerning illness and health care.

The composition, coverage, and operational trend of China's national medical security system

The national medical security system in China is a multilevel system, with the basic medical insurance (BMI) as the pillar and medical aid as the backup, and commercial health insurance, charitable donations, and medical mutual aid activities as supplementary services.

The BMI system serves two groups of people: employees and residents. Employees are enrolled in the employee basic medical insurance (EBMI) program, and non-working residents are enrolled in the residents basic medical insurance (RBMI) program. After being established in 2018, the National Healthcare Security Administration (NHSA) has continued to improve the national medical insurance system so that RBMI can be better integrated. As of September 2020, more than 1.35 billion people (over 95% of China's population) are covered by one of the BMI programs, making it the world's largest healthcare security network. The medical insurance fund is sustainable and growing. In 2019, the revenue of the national basic medical insurance fund (including maternity insurance) was CNY ¥2.44 trillion, and the expenditure was CNY ¥2.09 trillion [1].

Medical aid ensures all citizens have fair access to basic medical services by supporting the section of the low-income populace to participate in the BMI by subsidizing the medical expenses that they cannot afford. Since 2018, medical aid has benefited 480 million low-income citizens, helped reduce their medical burden by approximately CNY ¥330 billion, implemented targeted poverty reduction measures for 10 million people in need who were impoverished due to illnesses, and ensured their basic medical security. Various social forces in the market also actively participate in supplementing the medical security system and have become an important element of the multilevel medical insurance system.

Characteristics and advantages of China's healthcare security system

The Chinese government has always regarded people's health and life safety as its basic responsibility, by providing the BMI as a public good for all Chinese citizens. However, a deficit in coverage still exists between China and other countries with developed social security systems. The proportion of total medical insurance financing is about 2.5% of China's GDP, which is not high, but it is generally compatible with the per capita GDP of US $10,000 in China [2].

(I) Provide more. For one, government funding should be increased. From 2007 to 2019, government funding for medical security increased from CNY ¥91.3 billion CNY ¥800 billion, and the proportion of government spending on medical insurance increased from 1.87% to 3.50%. In 2020, the government subsidy for resident medical security reached CNY ¥550 per person [3]. For another, focus should remain on

守在生命的边缘
医者沉思录

the low-income population. Policies should lean towards the low-income population to ensure they have access to the BMI. The government continued to increase funding, and more than 99.9% of registered low-income citizens are now insured. The imbursement rate of hospitalization expenses has stabilized at around 80% for the low-income population after the broad coverage provided by the triple security system: the BMI, critical illness insurance, and medical aid [4].

(II)Stay within economic capabilities. To ensure the sustainable balance of the fund, financial overcommitment should be avoided, and the planning should be informed by the current level of economic development. The fund should meet the basic needs of people, but it should avoid becoming a welfare fund.

(III) Reinforcing the administration of the security system. First, a nationally organized volume-based procurement and use of drug standard should be established. A total of 112 types of drugs were procured by China in three batches, with the costs decreasing by an average of 54%, which saved CNY ¥53.9 billion annually [5]. Second, the catalog of medicines covered by the national health security system should be dynamically adjusted. Some obsolete drugs have been removed from the catalog to make room for drugs with more clinical value. Third, a reformation of medical insurance payment methods needs to be steadily implemented. In China, 97.5% of the local administrations have capped the total regional expense of medical insurance, and more than 30 pilot cities have launched diagnosis-related group payment systems. Fourth, medical organizations should be strictly supervised and unlawful practices should be heavily penalized. In the past 2 years, 330,000 unlawful organizations were suspended, and CNY ¥12.56 billion in funds were retrieved. In 2019, 69 inspection teams were sent to 30 provinces across the country to conduct unannounced field inspections, and CNY ¥2.232 billion in illegal funds were found.

Reforming the drug pricing mechanism and promoting drug availability for patients

The NHSA has implemented dynamic adjustments to the catalog of medicines covered by the national health security system and issued the *Interim Measures on the Administration of Medicines under the Basic Medical Insurance* [6]. The interim measures are oriented towards meeting the basic medicinal needs of citizens and ensuring that drug expenditures are compatible with BMI funding. It is necessary to ensure a scientific, standardized, precise, and dynamic management of medical insurance drugs. For exclusively produced drugs, the price is determined by catalog access negotiation, which not only saves medical insurance funds but also significantly reduces the burden of cost to patients. The establishment of a dynamic adjustment mechanism can facilitate the timely inclusion of more effective drugs into the catalog.

An example of this has been in the management of hepatitis-related drugs. In recent years, with the continuous efforts of the government, the price of drugs for viral hepatitis has been reduced substantially. In 2015, the annual treatment cost of hepatitis B antiviral drugs, tenofovir disoproxil fumarate (TDF) and entecavir, was about CNY ¥20,000 and CNY ¥9,000 per person, respectively. In 2018, after the "4+7" Pilot Program was launched, the annual treatment cost of TDF and entecavir was decreased to CNY ¥210-240 per person. In 2019, after more cities were included in the pilot program, the cost of the two drugs was further decreased to CNY ¥70. After the centralized procurement of entecavir, the total procurement volume was 3.5 times lower than that of the previous year in the "4+7" pilot cities. The same year, the NHSA also negotiated and reimbursed a variety of hepatitis C oral drugs, so the out-of-pocket costs paid by patients dropped by 95%. With the substantial reduction in drug prices, the diagnosis rate and the availability of chronic hepatitis treatment were considerably improved, which enabled China to achieve the 2030 Sustainable Development Goal outlined by the World Health Organization: eliminating hepatitis as a public health threat.

Building a multilevel medical security system to reinforce support capabilities

In recent years, China's commercial health insurance premium income has developed rapidly at an annual growth rate of 30%. In 2019, the premium income of commercial health insurance was CNY ¥706.6 billion, which represented a year-on-year increase of 29.7% [7]. To meet people's growing needs of health care in the new era, the government proposes to strengthen the triple security system, which includes basic medical insurance, critical illness insurance, and medical aid, and promote various complementary medical insurance programs for major and critical diseases. The development of commercial health insurance will be accelerated, more health insurance products will be offered, the individual income tax policies for commercial health insurance will be applied in a more effective way, and the scope of insurance products will be expanded [8].

Seizing opportunities, meeting challenges, and promoting the high-quality development of medical security

The year 2020 is the final year of *13th Five-Year Plan*, and it is also the year to lay a good foundation for the *14th Five-Year Plan*. Standing at this critical juncture, it is necessary to have a clear understanding of the challenges faced by health security.

The demographics of the Chinese population poses serious challenges to the sustainability of the fund. The number of people over the age of 60 will exceed 300 million people at the end of the *14th Five-Year Plan*, and the ratio of employees to retirees will continue to decline [9]. Another serious challenge is that communicable diseases and chronic diseases pose a "double burden" on China's medical insurance funds. There is still a gap between the healthcare security support and the medical expectations of citizens.

Medical security is highly relevant to the vital interests of the Chinese people as a whole. During the *14th Five-Year Plan* period, the government will continue to promote the integrity of the multilevel medical security and guide the coordinated development of medical security, treatment, and medicine, so that the people can have more clear and accountable expectations for their health security and a greater sense of gain, healthy security and happiness in turn.

References

［1］National Healthcare Security Development Report 2019. Available online: http://www.nhsa.gov.cn/art/2020/6/24/art_7_3268.html.

［2］What it means that the GDP per capita exceeds 10,000 US dollars. 2020. Available online: https://baijiahao.baidu.com/s?id=1656049179746010782&wfr=spider&for=pc.

［3］The Notice of Preparing Relevant Work of 2020 Residents Basic Medical Security, National Healthcare Security Administration, Ministry of Finance, State Taxation Administration. 2020. Available online: http://www.gov.cn/zhengce/zhengceku/2020-06/19/content_5520571.htm

［4］The "three-year action" of medical insurance poverty alleviation has reduced the burden of the poor by nearly 300 billion Yuan. 2020. Available online: http://www.xinhuanet.com/politics/2020-10/14/c_1126611738.htm.

［5］The state has made remarkable achievements in the centralized purchase of drugs, saving 53.9 billion yuan annually, and the average price of the purchased three batches of drugs has reduced more than half. 2020. Available online: http://sh.people.com.cn/n2/2020/1014/c138654-34348282.html.

［6］Interim measures for drug administration of basic medical insurance. 2020.

Available online: http://www.gov.cn/zhengce/zhengceku/2020-08/04/con-
tent_5532409.htm.

[7] Data from China Banking and Insurance Regulatory Commission. Available online: http://www.cbirc.gov.cn/cn/view/pages/index/index.html.

[8] Opinions on Deepening the Reform of Medical Security System, The CPC Central Committee, The State Council. 2020. Available online: http://www.gov.cn/
zhengce/2020-03/05/content_5487407.htm.

[9] Zheng Bingwen: China's elderly population will exceed 300 million at the end of
the 14th Five-Year Plan. 2020. Available online: http://bgimg.ce.cn/xwzx/gnsz/
gdxw/202010/27/t20201027_35939625.shtml.

主编导读（十九）

中医中药在现在医疗中的定位：中药会毁了中医吗？

这是一篇述评文章，有关中医中药对现代中国患者的疗效和作用。实际上我早就想涉足这个问题了，它在临床医疗上是一个现实且重要的问题，同时也是一个敏感的话题。

我个人对中医中药在临床上所扮演的角色也存在一种非常矛盾和复杂的感觉。从宏观上讲，中医中药是从整体的和哲学的观点去认识和看待疾病，这种整体观是现代科学发展方向之一。从历史数据看，我们中华民族的人口总数直到清朝末年，一直排在世界前列。不可否认，在西医引进中国之前，中医中药护佑了我们的先辈，是我们人口总数维持在世界第一的重要原因之一。

但是，我国医学界尤其是西医学界常常对中医中药有怀疑和不信任感。其一，有些患者在服用中药后出现了副作用，尤其是对于肝脏的损害。在手术后，经过中药调理的患者，有些会出现不同程度的药物性肝炎和肝损伤，这其中就包括我本人的亲朋好友，更有少数患者因中药造成的肝功能损害严重到不可恢复的程度，不得不进行肝移植。因此，我对肝脏外科手术后的患者服用中药是有点忌讳的。当然，这种现象是不是与现在的中药药材有关呢？我们已经不是李时珍爬悬崖采仙草的时代了，中药药材规模化的生产和销售，会不会带来质量上的不稳定或者充假现象？这些也是需要验证的问题。其二，中医中药迟迟不能实现"分子生物学机制化"过程，不能说服现代医学界那些越来越以精准医疗和循证医学的医生（不是中医的循证，而是循分子生物学机制之证）。在这些背景下，不仅西医界怀疑和质疑，连中医界也有朋友提出较激进的"别让中药毁了中医"的说法。

我与北京广安门中医院的吕文良院长每每谈到这些对于中医的抵触情绪的时候，哪怕是用最为温和、隐晦的语气说出，都会遭到吕院长的迎头痛斥，言辞抨击，他有一套很好的理论来说明和解释这个问题。所以我请他写了一篇相关的述评，来谈中医的理论和实践，当然也一定要谈到大家关心的问题和疑惑。

认识中医

吕文良

中国中医科学院广安门医院

中医学是传承数千年的生命科学，是一代代中华医者在临床与疾病斗争的过程中不断实践、总结再被验证、实践的科学认识，是中国古代科学和中华文化智慧的结晶。中医学由于其疗效的奇特性和可靠性引起了广泛的重视，但又由于其发展的不全面性及来自各界不同认识论的审视，受到了一些非议。

中医学的起源应该跟中国文化起源相同步，是中国传统文化孕育出的硕果。中医学相关的文字记载可追溯到先秦两汉时期，几千年以来，因为受各种条件的限制，我们只是从中医学自身完善的理论体系去阐述中医学对人体的认识和治病的机制。中医学的生命力在于临床疗效和安全性，历代医家在不断地传承发展它，在这个过程中许多宝贵的内容被传承了下来，也有部分遗失了，究其原因有许多。近现代以来随着国际社会的交流不断扩大和深化，西医学科学因其直观的线性思维及其疗效的客观可见，易于为大家所接受，主流医学界因此希望看到中医学也建立这样的体系，但事实上这个问题很难解决，难解决不等于不能解决，需要时间和耐心。现就以下几个中医学问题同大家探讨。

解读神明

《黄帝内经灵枢·天年》载："失神者死，得神者生也"，神是人生命活动客观规律的主宰，有元神、识神之分。医道同源互生，道家理论中相关论述可作参考。《玄肤论·元精元气元神论》云："所谓元神，非思虑之神之谓也，神通于无极，父母未生以前之灵真也"，元神与生俱来，为心所主；识神为后天所得，与所受的教育及社会环境有关，为脑所主。《医学衷中参西录·人身神明诠》又言："元神者，无思无虑，自然虚灵也。识神者，发于心，有思有虑，灵而不虚也"，论述了两者的功能特点，元神有主宰生命活动、化生统管五脏神之功，还可感通天地。（如行心脏置换术后的患者爱上心脏捐赠者的爱人现象等）。随着现代科技的不断进步，人们一方面对外物的学习运用愈加强化，另一方面，与生俱来的天分禀赋、对宇宙的感知能力却逐渐退化。正如法国生物学家拉马克提出的"用进废退"进化论，识神渐增而元神逐减，现代人对古人内修身心，通过感悟天地认知中医气血、经络、阴阳等的感受能力消退，对中医的认识能力随之下降。因此，加强对元神的锻炼和认识，是能够从精神层面感悟中医、解释中医疗效的一种途径。

认识物质

我们对事物的认识主要来自物质层面，而物质主要分三类：一类是视之有物，触之有形的，能够被直接测量和研究；一类是视之有物，触之无形，但能通过其他方式来验证研究的（如空气中的氧气通过氧化反应被证实存在）；还有一类视之无形，触之无形的，目前也难以验证的，但我们不能否定它的存在，如中医的经络，经络有名而无形，要通过练功去实现对它存在的研究。我们集中人力、物力，使用现行固有的意识形态去探索、研究未知物质的存在，这或许亦是宇宙目前许多难以解释的问题存在的原因，宇宙中一定存在着常人看不见也摸不着的未知物质，如暗物质等，一些科学家正努力研究证实它，如果从神学角度去理解、构思、研究，也许是另一种实现突破的途径。优秀的物理学家牛顿由物理学转而从事神学可能就是一个例子。总而言之，不能因为我们自身认识能力的局限性以及现存科学手段、客观设备无法验证未知物质，就否定它的存在。中医学对人体的认识正是基于以上三个层面综合展开的，因此比较难以被常人理解。

证实经络

中医理论的物质组成主要包括脏腑体系和经络体系两部分，《黄帝内经》对此有详细的阐述。经络是什么，是国内外一直在探究的热点问题。现在世界上很多国家都承认以经络穴位为基础的针灸疗法，是因为其具有显著的即时疗效。但目前对经络的研究，主要是从经络可视化、有形化、物质化的角度去进行的，这种研究存在两种缺陷：第一，将经络孤立于中医学自身的理论体系之外，采用的是违背中医学对人体经络认识的研究方法；第二，研究的主体对经络学（包括穴位）的本质没有任何自我实践，所以大量的经穴研究暂时都未取得实质的进展。

中医与中药

关于中医亡于中药的认识：首先，中医是一个综合的疗法，不仅利用中药来治病。中医学经典《黄帝内经》就分为《灵枢》和《素问》两个部分，分别以脏腑和经络为核心论述。我们在认识中医的过程中，除了中药治疗，还要考虑到中医的针灸、按摩、导引，包括祝由术、心理治疗等；其次是药物种植这部分。总体来说，由于人类社会的发展及特定资源的匮乏，我们生活生产方式发生了很大的变化。目前来说，虽然我们的食物是通过化肥、农药种植的，但能够满足人类对日常营养摄取的需要；我们的中药也面临着同样的情况，大部分中药都是通过种植获得，野生中药越来越少，这对其性味功能会有一些影响，虽然目前难以评价这些影响究竟有多大，但总归不是很危险。

中医亡于中药，最大的问题不在于中药的规模化种植，而是受到西方文化的影响太多。第一是动物保护组织对一些动物药的限制，比如，犀角是退热解毒、治血小板减少性紫癜特别好的药物，现在已经不能使用。第二是对中药毒性的认识不全面，导致现在国内很多医生都不再且不能使用有毒中药，这其实比第一点还更重要。第三与药物的质量有关。第四与药物的品种和地道性有关。这些对于中医的发展确实有着很大的影响。去年新冠病毒感染大流行时，产生了诸如"清肺排毒汤"等疗效显著的"三方"，这三个方剂里，麻黄起到主要作用，如果少了麻黄，那么"三方"的疗效就难以体现，但是西医中麻黄却是禁用的，这就是中西方文化认识的不同。所以说中医亡于中药之说有一定道理。我们现在经常说保护珍稀动物，使得许多动物药无法使用；而且有毒的中药也不能使用，那么只靠剩下正向作用的药物的话，就相当于原本"两条腿走路"的中医的只剩下一条腿在走，疗效肯定会受重大影响，这当然可以理解为中医亡于中药。

此外，我们要全面、客观地去认识有毒中药。中医的治疗是靠正向作用和反向作用来治病，比如人参补气，这是众所周知的；而大家认为大黄是泻下的，但实际上它的机制不是这么简单。我们前面也提到，毒药是以毒攻毒的，那么不能使用有毒中药，中医就没办法以毒攻毒了，如商陆是很好的利水的药物，因为它有微毒，现在就不敢再用了。还有对有毒中药剂量的掌控也要注意，在药典中对药物的剂量有了一定的要求，有的是3克，有的是6～9克等。临床上，药物的使用剂量就如同饮酒，有的人酒量大，有的人酒量小，现在对药物的剂量加以限制，那么对不同程度的疾病，对不同的患者，就达不到有效剂量。如果达不到治疗剂量的话，就没有疗效，达到治疗剂量的话，就有可能中毒，这是一个要全面去认识的问题。

中药与毒性

有部分中药有毒，但炮制和复方可以减毒增效。以何首乌为例，这几年有关何首乌肝毒性的报道非常之多，302医院的肖小河教授研究后发现：何首乌不能跟铁器放在一起煎煮，它能把二价铁变成三价铁，而三价铁对肝肾的毒性是非常大的。我查阅古代医籍，发现古人对何首乌的应用提出了两点：第一个就要忌铁器，第二个要跟黑豆一起去炮制，九蒸九晒去解毒；由此可见，古人虽然不知道药物毒性的机制在哪，但是已经找到制约药物毒性的答案。那么除了何首乌要忌铁器，其他药物要不要忌铁器呢？于是我想到小时候就听说煎药不能用铁锅煎，在西藏用银碗银筷，现在知道原因了。先人就是通过这样一种方法来解决药物的毒性问题。因此我们对中药的毒性要有全面、正确的认识，第一要考虑以毒攻毒，第二要考虑药物在炮制以后、在合理的组方以后就没有毒性了。对中药的肝毒性要有客观的评价，就像肿瘤患者应用的化疗药物，尽管化疗药物对人体的肝脏、肾脏、血液系统、骨髓等功能都有损伤，但因为要治疗肿瘤，只能两害相权取其轻，继续使用。

中医与西医

大家普遍认为中医是整体的、宏观的、辩证的，西医是具体的、微观的、科学的。但在我看来，中西医的主要差别不在这里，而在于中医认识人体和疾病时，是始终把物质和精神统一起来，不是割裂来看的，并且中医关注"天时地利"等社会生活环境因素对人体和疾病的影响，而西医主要是从解剖层面（物质）来认识人体。具体体现在中医与西医对疾病的认识上：中医使用统一的证候理论来指导临床方药的使用，证候学正是一个中医方剂可以治不同疾病的理论基础；而西医的认识是以病为基础，什么药治什么病，并且在这一套理论的指导下形成了一个相对固态的思维，因此在发展过程中容易创造一些引起医学界轰动的成绩，比如西地那非原本用于研究治疗心血管疾病，后来被发现可以应用于男性性功能障碍；再比如黄连素（小檗碱）被发现还可以用于降血糖。但是对中医来说，这只是很简单的异病同治思想的一个体现，没有那么复杂。从矛盾的角度看，西医更多解决的是矛盾的普遍性，相对而言结合个人临床经验较少，千篇一律的标准化疗效很好，但是难以解决特殊的疾病；而中医的思维方法既能够解决矛盾的普遍性，又能解决特殊性，这是中医疗效全面、安全确切的基础之一。

中医和西医对疾病的认识发展也取决于两个主体中个人的综合素养。西医大夫可以站在巨人的肩膀上去解决一些问题，而对中医大夫来说却不可能，任何中医大夫都是从零开始，从头学起，这也是大家说中医学是经验医学的原因。治一些别人治不好的病，成为一个优秀的中医生，不仅需要建立在个人后天努力学习，有一定的学科理解的基础（即基于识神发挥作用的基础上），不断积累临床经验，还要充分发挥对生命的感知能力（元神的作用）。

诊疗标准

中医学的理论体系形成与中国古代哲学是相辅相成的，它追求的是人体阴阳五行的平衡、同时与宇宙的和谐共存。不管人体处于什么年龄阶段，首先要保持人体的脏腑、气血、阴阳的平衡。所以中医在治病的过程中，不仅注重对致病原因（病因）的治疗，如外感病的祛邪疗法（如清热解毒、活血利水法等），内伤病的扶正疗法（健脾益肾、柔肝养心等）；还会使用各种治疗手段，使人体的各个器官组织协调发挥其最大的作用（整体观念），这也是中医治疗患病机体最主要的一个特点。

中医学在治疗中重视运用综合治疗手段激活、提高、发挥机体的自我调节功能（自愈能力），这是西医学临床中往往会忽略的，这种忽略反映了现在西医学科划分过细的一些问题。西医有研究发现一个疾病在进行专科治疗的同时，如果加以免疫治疗，疗效较佳，他们认为这是一种很高明的办法，但在中医学体系中却是一种最常见的治疗思想，这也是中医治疗中出现诸多奇特疗效个案的原因，也是中医学被神化的主要因素之一。正是中医学治疗方法、治疗手段、治疗理念这三条作用途径同时发挥作用才造就了中医疗效的神奇性。同时又因为各医家对疾病不同层次的认识和经验，加之每个患者自身体质的不同，往往造成同一个中医生针对同一种疾病的不同个体无法实现现代医学研究过程中所谓的"临床疗效的可重复性"，这是下一步中医学界要解决的问题，因此说用标准化来衡量疗效或确定治疗方案，只能解决矛盾的普遍性，不能解决特殊性，事实上目前西医重视个体化治疗正是向中医靠拢。中医体系的标准化由四诊合参，经络、脏腑、八纲辨证等诊疗标准构成，不能够用中医疗效的不可重复性和能否实现现代医学意义的标准化来衡量评价中医，妖魔化中医。

中医学的发展确实遇到了很多问题，但中医自信是建立在我们临床疗效的基础上的。至于对中医的研究，首先不能违背中医的自身发展规律，其次，建议大家去切身感受一下，尤其是对经络的认识，没有实践就没有发言权，这个实践是要全面的、具体的、长期的、不带偏见的。

Understanding traditional Chinese medicine

Lv Wenliang

Guanganmen Hospital, China Academy of Chinese Medical Sciences,
Beijing, China

Traditional Chinese Medicine (TCM), a collection of ancient Chinese knowledge and cultural wisdom, is a life science that has been passed down for thousands of years. Supporters of TCM stress its clinical efficacy, and while the particular characteristics and reliability of TCM have received widespread attention, they have also invited considerable criticism. This article aims to discuss some of these controversial topics.

Decipher the spirit—Shen

Shen is the basis for all human activities and the source from which all human spirit emerges. *Shen* can be divided into soul and wisdom. The soul is inborn, and it is contained in the heart—the "monarch"—of all human organs. Thus, practitioners of TCM believe that the heart can govern all life activities via other organs and perceive external feedback. For example, a patient who has received a heart transplant may fall in love with the heart donor's lover—because the soul is governed by the heart. Wisdom is acquired, and it is contained in the brain. With the development of modern science and technology, people can learn new subjects much faster and deepen their wisdom, but their souls—the innate ability to perceive the universe—have gradually deteriorated. The balance between the soul and wisdom has been tilted so askew that it has become harder for people to perceive *Yin* and *Yang*, *Qi* (energy) and blood in

TCM. Physicians in TCM must not only accrue clinical experience and accumulate wisdom, but also increase their awareness to perceive life and nature (the soul).

Understand substances

Our understanding of substances is mainly based on their appearances. Some substances are tangible, and some are intangible. The intangible can be further divided into verifiable substances (such as oxygen) and unverifiable substances, such as meridians in TCM. Meridians are intangible, but their existence can be sensed through clinical practice. There are still many unknown substances in the universe that have yet to be discovered and verified. A good approach to these unknown substances is to learn through theology. An example of this is can be found in the life of Sir Isaac Newton. His research interest spanned both the subjects of physics and theology, as theology is another way to acquire insights into the workings of the universe. In short, people should be aware that simply because the existence of an object has yet to be proven, it does not mean the object does not exist.

It is generally believed that TCM is holistic, macroscopic, and dialectical, while Western medicine is specific, microscopic, and scientific. However, in my opinion, the main difference between Chinese and Western medicine is that Chinese medicine attempts to unify the material and the spiritual, and it considers the influence of social and environmental factors, such as time and location, on the human body and diseases; meanwhile, Western medicine mainly considers the human body on the anatomical level (material level).

Verification of meridians

TCM theory is composed of two principal parts: the solid viscera system and the meridian system, which are explained in detail in the

Inner Canon of the Yellow Emperor (*also known as Huangdi Neijing*). The practice of acupuncture, in which the therapist inserts needles into acupoints under the skin, is widely accepted across the globe, as it can improve the quality of life of the patient. Acupoints are located on meridians, which are the 12 pathways in the body that connect vital organs, allowing energy to flow through. However, current research on meridians mainly focuses on the visual, tangible, and material aspects of meridians, which is problematic for 2 reasons: first, it neglects the holistic nature of the TCM by isolating meridians from other influence factors and thereby violates the principles of TCM research; second, many researchers have little experience in practicing the essence of the meridian, and so a large number of meridian and acupoint studies fail to make substantial progress.

Standards of diagnosis and treatment

The formation of the TCM theoretical system is consonant with ancient Chinese philosophy. It pursues the balance between the *Yin* and *Yang*, between the *Five Elements* of the human body, and the harmonious coexistence of humanity with the universe. Regardless of one's age or gender, the balance of the *Yin* and *Yang* in one's viscera, *Qi* (energy) and blood is vital. For exogenous disease causes, TCM physicians remove disease-causing factors and treat the condition accordingly (which may include detoxification, heatstroke cooling, promoting blood circulation and diuresis, etc.); for internal injuries, TCM strengthens the organs' vitality (nourishing the heart, protecting the liver, invigorating the spleen and kidney, etc.). Therefore, when treating a patient, TCM not only treats the underlying causes of diseases, but also coordinates the organs and tissues of the human body to facilitate its maximum capacity for recovery (holistic therapy). TCM attaches great importance to the use of comprehensive treatment to activate, improve, and exert the body's self-regulation function (self-healing ability). This integration of the whole body's function is often neglected in the clinical practice of Western medicine because of its current fragmentation into various subspecialties and its conceptual division of the human body into specific organs and corresponding diseases. Western medicine has recently discovered that immunotherapy is an effective treatment for some patients, but this theory has been widely accepted in TCM therapy for quite some time. The concept of immunotherapy can also explain the peculiar cases of curative recovery in TCM, the occurrence of which is one of the main factors contributing to the veneration of TCM. It is precisely the coordination of treatment concepts and methods that creates the miraculous effects sometimes seen in TCM. However, because different doctors have different levels of understanding and experience with diseases, and because each patient is unique, a TCM practitioner may often fail to achieve the so called "repeatability" of a clinical curative effect even for identical symptoms and diseases. This is a critical issue for TCM to solve going forward because the use of guidelines or standardized treatment can only be applied to determine the outcome of patients in general and not specific individuals. Interestingly, however, Western medicine has recently shifted focus to individualized treatment plans, which is more in line with tenets of Chinese medicine.

The standardization of the TCM consists of the four diagnostic methods, meridians, viscera, and the eight-principal syndrome differentiation. The efficacy of TCM should not be denied based on its lack of repeatability, nor should it be measured under the standard of modern medical science and dismissed thereby. TCM observes syndromes to guide clinical treatment, and part of the theoretical basis of the TCM is that a given prescription can be used to treat different diseases. Western medicine tends to build guidelines centering around a single specific disease, which is followed by standardized medicine and treatment plans. During the development of Western medicine, the accidental use of a medicine beyond the intended scope of the guidelines occasionally produced surprising results. For example, sildenafil was originally used for the research and treatment of cardiovascular diseases but was later found to be applicable to male sexual dysfunction. In another example, it was found that berberine, an antidiarrheal drug, could also be used to lower blood sugar. Within the frame of TCM, these findings are not surprising, as they merely realize the concept of treating different diseases with the same methods. Indeed, this is the foundation of TCM—comprehensive, individualized, and systematic.

The development of the TCM has indeed encountered many difficulties, but we should maintain confidence in TCM based on its clinical efficacy. When conducting research into Chinese medicine, researchers should follow the principles and the naturalistic development pattern of TCM. Furthermore, real-world experience with acupuncture and meridians is needed to understand authentic TCM and to draw accurate conclusions regarding its efficacy. These conclusions should be comprehensive, precise, enduring, and unbiased.

主编导读（二十）

互联网医疗：可持续发展、能担当重任吗?

记得十多年以前，互联网医疗雏形是网上医疗咨询，到目前还有一些方兴未艾的医疗咨询网站，给患者和医生搭建了一个交流平台。这样，患者可以不用去医院挂号看病，有机会在线上直接咨询一些不太复杂的病症，这个确实为双方带来了很大的便利，不少基础疾病问题可以在线上解决，而且医生可以利用自己的碎片时间来完成这种咨询。我本人至今也通过这些平台线上答复患者的咨询和提问。

但当时想，所谓"网上看病"也就到此作为一个度了。因为内心不敢忘记并且笃信的是医学前辈们的经典原则，就是如果要诊治疾病，医生必须亲自仔细地接触、询问、检查患者，得到第一手材料，也就是中医学强调的"望闻问切"过程，才能负责地作出诊断，并制定治疗方案。前辈们还说了，现在的年轻医生不能光依赖化验单和影像检查结果下医学结论，忽视患者的面诊和体检程序，因为看病是一个复杂的综合信息的认知和判断过程。

至今我深感前辈的理念还是非常正确的。但是这样的话，互联网医疗还有后续发展吗? 所以当时很多人的理念是所谓互联网医疗也就是一个简单疾病的简单咨询、简单解答的事情。要再进一步深入，有可能会"出事情"了，甚至会有医疗事故。而真有事情的话，其中医疗责任的界定也会是一个问题。但是科学的发展总是出乎很多人的意料，俗定的规则也总是被一次次打破。就像18世纪初，如果有人说以后一个铁皮壳子能够在天上飞行，到达目的地，那一定会被认为是疯子，事到如今谁看到在空中飞行的飞机都习以为常了。在当今年代，互联网的高速发展，5G技术的广泛应用，人们对于网络上解决问题的习惯和信赖，已经打破了原来的经典框架，一切发生了耳目一新的变化。

现在，在网络上就诊看病、线上MDT大会诊甚至线上开处方都已经渐渐地成为现实。不久以前国内还把网络医疗发展成"互联网医院"，并且逐渐推广发展。对此我虽有耳闻但是了解有限，直到一次全国会议，有幸聆听了国内互联网医院的开创者和掌门人之一——复旦大学华山医院的张群华院长的报告，才领悟到国内的网上医疗已经发展到如此发达的地步了。

对于张群华院长的报告比较深刻的印象是，互联网医疗实际上起步于西方，但是真正高速发展的却是在中国（如同许多行业，只要国外一创新，就有人搬到国内来，然后做到极致），在互联网医疗方面国内是真正的弯道超车。这个现象一方面得益于中国的网络技术普及惊人地快，也被广大民众所接受和认可；另一方面是新冠病毒感染疫情，新冠病毒感染疫情带来很多健康和社会问题，但是也正是这个时候，互联网医疗彰显出它的优势来，使它得以更快地发展和普及。

即使是这样，我心里还是有小小的疙瘩的。因为很多快速兴起的新兴产业经过一段时间耀眼的发展后，又慢慢消停下来或者降到一个应该有的热度（如共享单车或者共享汽车），那么互联网医疗到底最后会发展到什么地步呢？它会有可持续的发展吗？能不能真正在医疗领域里担当起一个的主要角色呢？为此我专门请教了张群华院长，他谈了很多，让我耳目一新，我就此邀请他写下这篇有关互联网医疗的文章。

中国互联网医疗方兴未艾

张群华

复旦大学上海华山医院

互联网医疗在中国已经普及。2015年12月，由微医创办的乌镇互联网医院成为中国首家互联网医院，开启了互联网医疗的新篇章。特别是2019年新冠疫情的出现，中国互联网医院进入了快速发展的轨道。截至2021年6月，中国已有1600家互联网医院，他们在中国形成了门诊、住院和线上三位一体的新颖医疗模式。极大地方便了患者就医，有效地提高了医生的工作效率，缓解了中国优质医疗资源的短缺现状。

欧美等国互联网医疗先行一步

随着1991年互联网的第一个web服务器斯坦福线性加速器（SLAC）的创建和1992互联网平台的大量注册，奠定了"互联网＋医疗服务"的基础。进入21世纪后，web2.0和web3.0为互联网医疗服务创造了快速发展条件。3G/4G以及其他新技术促进互联网医疗快速发展。美国凯撒医疗集团的互联网医疗发展很迅速，52%的初诊通过在线完成。78%的美国家庭医生认为通过互联网医疗可以提高诊断质量和就医渠道。而且在美国，家庭医生作为线上线下融合纽带可加速互联网医疗转诊水平，67%的患者认为互联网医疗提高了就诊满意度。日本最近兴起一股"在线诊疗"的热潮，数字医疗有助降低成本，2021年日本使用数字化医疗机构所占比例上升至15%。英国互联网医疗服务分为基于国家层面的国家互联网医疗服务系统，基于地区的互联网医疗初级医疗健康系统，基于日益增长的自我健康管理和护理需求的解决方案系统。国外互联网医疗起步早，各国发展都依据本国医疗供需采用的互联网模式各异，其中利弊值得借鉴和学习。

我国互联网医疗弯道超车

鉴于我国医疗长期面临供需矛盾突出的根本性问题。人口老龄化加剧，慢病患者增多，人们健康意识增强，医疗消费幅度增长，催生了大量的医疗需求。从供给端来讲我国优质医疗资源不足，且资源分布不均，难以满足增长的需求。随着移动互联网的快速发展催生了新的医疗健康信息化服务模式。2010年前后，在我国相继出现了丁香园、好大夫在线、春雨医生、挂号网等平台。应用模式分为面向医生、面向用户与患者两种模式。部分公立医院推出掌上医院，集中在健康咨询服务、图文问诊、门诊精准预约、远程视频会诊、医患交流等方面。2015年12月乌镇互联网医院作为全国首家互联网医院创建于第二届世界互联网大会期间，乌镇互联网医院的创新发展有四个方面：①互联网医院首先是医疗实体，也是线上诊治的责任主体；②互联网医院只开展复诊和远程会诊，减少了医疗风险；③互联网医院可以让医生多点执业，有利于患者找对医生；④互联网医院可以开电子处方，医生在互联网医院注册备案，并且每一张处方有药剂师审核。由此互联网医院打破了时空限制，互联网医疗进入1.0时代，开辟了数字医疗新路径。

2018年国家出台新政策，强调积极发展"互联网＋医疗健康"，开展预约诊疗、慢病复诊、远程医疗等线上服务。允许依托医疗机构发展互联网医院，医疗机构可以使用互联网医院作为第二名称，在实体医院基础上应用互联网技术提供安全适宜的医疗服务。2021年3月"互联网＋医疗服务"的医保支付政策与线下一致，标志着中国互联网医疗发展进入2.0新阶段，形成了以政府为主导，公立医院为主体，企业互联网医院参与的新格局。

新冠疫情使互联网医疗迎来高光时刻

2019年全球出现了新冠疫情，此次疫情在一定程度上倒逼中国

守在生命的边缘
医者沉思录

医疗卫生服务能力的提升。基于病毒传染性极强的特点，各医疗机构逐步上线了互联网医疗服务，尽量减少医患直接接触的机会。这种新的诊疗模式，促使了医疗服务模式从面对面医疗向线上线下相结合转变。医疗服务场所也从医院进一步延伸，覆盖患者全生命周期，有助于建立慢性病分级防治体系，以及患者一体化全面管理体系。疫情防控期间，医院线上的门诊量、互联网平台的咨询量都呈现爆发式增长。大众仿佛一夜之间就接受了网上看病的模式，疫情催生了大量的互联网医疗的红利。据中国社科院健康事业发展研究中心统计，中国有644.9亿次的患者浏览轨迹，6.8亿次医患交流，7409万的患者互联网医疗服务。仅复旦大学附属华山医院皮肤科，网上访问量累计达1亿次，在线服务患者累计超过23万；上海儿童医学中心，网上的总浏览量已经达到3.41亿次，该院80%以上的主治医生开通了互联网医疗平台。上海儿童医学中心院长张浩教授是一名小儿外科医生，在互联网平台上服务了6100名患者，有360万的点击量。他认为，医生、医院要在互联网上抢占先机。在新冠疫情后，他觉得真正进入了互联网医疗的春天。微医、好大夫在线、丁香园、京东健康、平安好医生等在新冠疫情期间承接了众多慢性病和肿瘤患者的咨询及复诊，发挥了积极作用。

线上线下医疗质量同质化

截至2021年6月，中国互联网医院已经超过1600多家，实现了互联网医院与线下医院服务同质化迫在眉睫。国家出台政策要求互联网医疗平台所有电子处方、相关的记录，均应可追溯，并向省级监管平台开放数据接口。其次，平台内部必须有专职管理医疗质量安全、药学服务、信息技术等的部门。最后，防止药品销售平台将互联网诊疗变成营销工具。在疫情防控期间，北京大学肿瘤医院的互联网诊疗量占线下门诊量的30%，患者端、线上线下一体化就诊基本形成；广东省中医院互联网医院推出"在线医保复诊"便民功能，慢性病患者在家复诊开药，还能医保报销；首都医科大学天坛医院正在打造门诊患者线上化、住院患者连续化、外地患者集约化、线上专家批量化、预约门诊智能化的互联网诊疗平台。

我国互联网医疗进入3.0时代

如今互联网医疗已经进入3.0时代，标志着随着5G技术和人工智能技术的介入，互联网医疗呈现规模化、常态化和智能化。中日友好医院互联网医院已连通全国6000家医疗机构，包括580家医养结合机构，实施了31.3万例远程会诊，有效解决了偏远地区疑难病患者就诊难问题。慢病专科管理成为互联网医疗的新趋势；上海瑞金医院牵头，联合多家企业创建了国家标准化代谢性疾病管理中心（the National Metabolic Management Center，MMC），应用了人工智能、物联网、大数据等新技术，全国有近1500家医院加入MMC行列，共管理80万糖尿病患者。这80万患者的糖化达标率（HbA1c<7%）从基线18.65%显著提升至45.46%，代谢指标的综合率从基线6.20%显著提升至17.94%（欧美均值14%）。糖尿病导致的血管、眼、肾、足等多个器官的并发症已实现大幅减少。在山东省泰安市，微医推行"互联网＋医联体"模式的慢病管理，通过数字化、规范化的全流程管理，强化了医保的监管和控费。当地慢性病患者人均就诊时间从2小时下降到30分钟，单次处方费用也降低了12.7%，让患者足不出户就能实现复诊购药；清华大学长庚医院董家鸿院士在北京利用5G互联网技术指导相距2200多公里的深圳市人民医院完成复杂肝脏肿瘤手术。

可喜的是截至2021年12月，中国网民规模达到10.32亿，互联网普及率达到73.0%，使用手机上网的比例达99.7%。在线医疗用户规模达2.98亿，同比增长了38.7%。国家卫生健康委《医疗机构设置规划指导原则》（2021－2025年）指出，大力发展互联网诊疗服务，形成线上线下一体化服务模式，提高医疗服务体系整体效能。由此可见，我国互联网医疗正处于方兴未艾的时期。

The internet hospital: how to combine with traditional healthcare model

Zhang Qunhua

Huashan Hospital, Fudan University, Shanghai, China

The development of online health services in the world

The history of the internet hospital could be traced back to 1991, when the Stanford Linear Accelerator Center (SLAC) began to host the first World Wide Web server (web1.0). In 1992, a large number of internet platforms were registered, which laid the groundwork for "online + offline" health services. Entering the 21st century, the modified web server (web2.0 and web3.0) provided the possibility for the rapid development of internet hospitals. In addition, the 3G/4G network and other new technologies promoted the expansion of internet hospitals. In the United States, the online health service of Kaiser Permanent (an American integrated managed care consortium) was quite mature, with 52% of the patient's first doctor visits being completed online. Family physicians often play a key role between online and offline medical services conversion, and about 78% of American family physicians believed that online health services can provide alternative access to healthcare and improve patients' healthcare quality. About 67% of the patient believed the online health services improved their level of satisfaction with doctor visits. In Japan, there was a boom in the number of internet hospitals recently. The percentile of Japanese hospitals that utilize digital healthcare system increased to 15% in 2021, because digitalization help reduces their medical costs. In the UK, the online medical services were divided into the national health system (NHS) for all citizens and the regional NHS for each geographic area, based on the needs of self-care and health management of its people. Overall, each system has its own advantages and disadvantages, and it is worth learning from one another.

The development of online health services in China

In recent years, internet hospitals have gradually become accessible in China. In December 2015, Wuzhen Internet Hospital was launched. Founded by WeDoctor (a Chinese online healthcare solutions platform), Wuzhen Internet Hospital was the first internet hospital in China, marking the beginning of Chinese online healthcare. In 2019, with the outbreak of the COVID-19 pandemic, Chinese internet hospitals have entered a period of rapid expansion. As of June 2021, there were 1,600 internet hospitals in China. Combining outpatient, inpatient and online healthcare three-in-one established an innovative healthcare model. It greatly assisted patients receiving medical treatment, improved doctors' efficiency, and relieved the burden of advanced healthcare resources in China.

Societal aging increased the number of patients with chronic diseases in China, so the medical costs and medical needs also largely built up. However, high-quality medical resources in China were insufficient and unevenly distributed, resulting in a deficit of people's increasing medical demands. The rapid development of mobile internet filled the deficit by generating a new digitalization healthcare service model. Around 2010, online network services such as DXY, Haodafu Online and Chunyu YiSheng subsequently appeared. These services have two categories: doctor-oriented (business-to-business) and patient-oriented (business-to-customer). Some public hospitals have launched "hand-held hospitals", which provide assistance in general health consultations, graphic or text consultations, outpatient appointments, telemedicine,

守在生命的边缘
医者沉思录

doctor-patient communications, and so on. As the first Internet hospital in China, Wuzhen Internet Hospital was founded during the Second World Internet Conference in December 2015. Wuzhen Internet Hospital has four innovations: (I) The internet hospital is an independent medical entity that acts as the main body for all online healthcare services. (II) The internet hospital only receives follow-up visits and remote consultations, reducing possible medical negligence and risks. (III) The internet hospital allows doctors to practice in multiple places, which also helps patients to find a satisfying doctor-patient relationship. (IV) Each doctor in the internet hospital is registered and filed, and each prescription is reviewed by a pharmacist. This combination breaks the constraints of time and space by issuing electronic prescriptions to patients, opening up a new route for digital healthcare.

In 2018, China began to actively develop "internet + medical health" system, providing online services such as doctor visit appointments, chronic disease follow-up, and telehealth. Organizations can rely on medical institution entities to establish internet hospitals and to supply the patient with safe and appropriate online medical services. In March 2021, the internet hospital health insurance payment policy was in line with the offline policy, entering a generation 2.0 of online health services. A new healthcare pattern, led by the government, public hospitals as the main body, with the cooperation of internet hospitals has been formed.

The COVID-19 pandemic prompted the internet hospital transformation

The global COVID-19 pandemic outbreak somehow forced the Chinese healthcare services to improve. Because the virus was highly contagious, numerous medical institutions have gradually launched online health services to minimize direct contact between doctors and patients, which prompt the transformation of the healthcare services from "face-to-face" to "online-offline mode". Healthcare locations were also further extended from hospitals only, to cover the prevention, treatment and rehabilitation of patients. All of these transformations helped to establish a hierarchical healthcare system for patients with chronic diseases and an integrated healthcare system for all patients. During the pandemic, the number of online outpatients' visits, and mobile platform consultations have grown exponentially. People were seen to have accepted online hospital visits overnight, which brought a huge bonus to the development of the internet hospital. According to the statistics from the Health Development Research Center of the Chinese Academy of Social Sciences, there were 64.49 billion times of patient browsing, 680 million times of doctor-patient communications, and 74.09 million times of online healthcare services for patients. The dermatology department of Huashan Hospital alone had accumulated 100 million times of online visits and served more than 230,000 patients online. In Shanghai Children's Medical Center, the total number of page views reached 341 million times, and more than 80% of the hospital attending doctors have opened their accounts on the online healthcare platform. The hospital's president, Professor Hao Zhang, is a pediatric surgeon who has served 6,100 patients on the online platform, with 3,6 million hits. He insists that doctors and hospitals should be pro-active on the internet. The spring of online healthcare will come after COVID-19. Online healthcare platforms like WeDoctor, Haodafu Online, DXY, Jingdong Health, and Ping An Good Doctor played an active role in patient follow-up with chronic diseases and tumors during the pandemic.

Unification of online and offline healthcare services

As of June 2021, there were more than 1,600 internet hospitals in China, and the unification of online and offline healthcare services is imminent. First, China required that all internet hospitals should have tracible electronic prescriptions and relevant medical records, with opening data access to provincial regulatory organizations. Secondly, internet hospitals must have a full-time department to supervise medical quality and safety, pharmaceutical services, information technology, etc. Third, avoiding drug sales companies from turning internet hospitals into marketing tools. During the pandemic, the online appointment visit accounted for 30% of the offline outpatient volume at Beijing Cancer Hospital. The Internet Hospital of Guangdong Traditional Chinese Medicine Hospital introduced an "online revisiting" service, allowing patients with chronic disease to follow-up and prescribe medicine at home with health insurance reimbursement. Beijing Tiantan Hospital of Capital Medical University created a healthcare platform that provides online services for outpatients, continuous healthcare for inpatients, resources centralization for non-local patients, gathering experts for remote consultation, an intelligent system for outpatient appointments, etc.

The internet hospital has entered generation 3.0. Online healthcare services have become more accessible, more popular and smarter with the help of the 5G network and artificial intelligence technology. The Internet Hospital of China-Japan Friendship Hospital has connected 6,000 medical institutions across the country, including 580 nursing homes. They held 313,000 times of telehealth consultations, effectively reducing the difficulty for patients from distant areas to receive adequate healthcare services. Specialist management of chronic diseases has become a new goal in the internet hospital. Shanghai Ruijin Hospital took the lead and cooperated with multiple companies to establish the National Metabolic Management Center (MMC). Nearly 1,500 hospitals across the country have joined the MMC to managed 800,000 diabetes patients through technologies like artificial intelligence, the Internet of Things, big data, etc. Among the 800,000 patients, the glycation compliance rate (HbA1c $< 7\%$) increased significantly from 18.65% to 45.46%, and the metabolic indicators increased significantly from 6.20.% to 17.94% (14% in Europe and America). Diabetic complications of vasculature, eyes, kidneys, feet and other organs were greatly reduced. In Tai'an, Shandong, WeDoctor implemented the "internet + integrated healthcare system" for chronic disease management. Through digitalized and standardized whole-process management, it strengthened the supervision of medical insurance. The average visiting time for local chronic disease patients has dropped from two hours to 30 minutes and the prescription cost was also reduced by 12.7% per time, allowing patients to refill medicines without leaving their homes. Professor Dong Jiahong from Beijing Tsinghua Changgung Hospital used the 5G network + mixed reality (MR) technology to guide complicated liver tumor surgery in Shenzhen People's Hospital, which is located 2,200 kilometers apart, indicating that the 5G network will bring infinite possibilities to online healthcare services.

As of December 2021, the population of Chinese netizens has reached 1.032 billion and the internet prevalence rate has reached 73.0%, with 99.7% of them being mobile phone users. The number of online healthcare users has reached 298 million, increasing by 38.7% per year. The National Health Commission's "Guiding Principles for the Planning of Medical Institutions (2021－2025)" pointed out that China should vigorously develop online healthcare services, form an integrated online and offline service model, and improve the overall efficiency of the healthcare system. Afterall, the future of Chinese online healthcare system is promising.

主编导读（二十一）

"信息化"时代的医学教育，老教授、病例和图书馆还能被称为"三件宝"吗？

北京协和医院"三件宝"，还剩几件？

我本人刚刚进入协和的时候，被反复传颂协和的"三件宝"，即老教授、病历和图书馆。协和之所以成为协和，保持和发扬这"三件宝"至关重要，后辈应该传承并且发扬光大。

实际上这在当年不无道理。早年协和的老教授占据了国内医学界各个领域的高峰，是学界的领头羊。中华医学会最初分学组分会的时候，一大部分分会的主委是协和的老教授。不仅如此，协和老教授还起到了难能可贵的承接中外交流的桥梁和纽带的作用。因为早年的协和以英语教学，又有各种天然的学术关系，使得在我国医学事业还处于相对落后的年代里，协和的老教授常常把国际领先的技术和理念带回中国，对于我国的医疗事业作出了显著的贡献。但是事到如今，全国各地学术界名师高徒辈出，和各国的交往已经非常广泛而深刻，协和的那些新一代"老教授"们已经不担负这些作用了。国内医学发展到今天，这些局面也是应该出现的现象。

规范的病历写作也曾经是协和的一大特点。在病案室里，你能查到民国早期各名人的病历，这些病历都作为原始资料保存了下来，供医生、学者查考，尤其珍贵。例如孙中山先生的病史和最后的病理解剖结果都在协和，坊间包括各种正式报道都认为孙中山先生是得肝癌去世的，但是我有幸看到原始病理报告，是一个法国医生用英文写的手写体，明明写着"胆囊癌肝转移"。这些材料有时揭示了一段历史，在病历书写完全手工化的年代里尤其难能可贵。但是现在病历已经完全电子化了。那些历史还是历史，但已经不可能重复出这些"历史"了。

图书馆是最为明显的变化，当年中国医学科学院（就是协和医学院）的图书馆是国内第二大医学图书馆，里面的馆藏非常珍贵而丰富，很多医学杂志在国内是孤本，常常看到"外地"医生，为了考证学术上某个说法、查找某个说法出处，连夜坐火车进京，找到协和图书馆，递上单位介绍信，在图书馆如饥似渴地查阅（越来之不易的就越是珍惜）。但是现在查阅文献已经完全电子化了，不要说去外地图书馆，就是图书馆在隔壁也不用去了，在网上一查，文献来得又快又全。这是非常伟大的进步。现在，有很多新的医学知识还靠微信公众号来传播；一个美国的年轻科学家告诉我，他很多新的专业界内容是从推特（Twitter，美国社交APP）上被推送得知的，因为推送的总是与你研究领域相关的研究成果，甚至连美国国立医学图书馆（Medline）都查得不多了。

那么从现在角度看，协和医院的"三件宝"还剩下几件宝呢？老教授（50后、60后）已经远远不是原来意义上的"协和老教授"了；病历档案原来的还在，还是起到见证历史的作用，但是已经不靠这些资料来"总结病例"和发表学术论文了，因为论文的性质、构架和目的也有了很大的改变；图书馆里纸板的杂志期刊更是被电子版的文章和查询工具所替代了。前不久英国外科杂志（*Brit J Surg*）发表声明，这本持续了一百多年的曾经是世界上最好的外科期刊，终于停止了印刷版，全部改为电子版了。

那么协和"三件宝"没有作用了吗？我认为还是有的，只是不那么具体化了。协和三件宝最后成为一个标志，来说明协和的医德、医风、医术的传承。这种传承非常难能可贵，不得不承认的一个事实是年轻医生从小在协和成长，他们的风格和素质本身就会不一样。"三件宝"已经从具体化变成了一种精神和传承，它可能是十件宝、几十件宝的一个缩影。

我想最应该评论这"三件宝"的应该是协和"亲生"的子弟，又在其他医院工作过，有了协和基因又有外面的视野。所以这次邀请了我们2004级北京协和医科大学八年制学长傅麒宁来对此问题进行评论，他目前在重庆高就。

协和三宝，风采能否依旧?

傅麒宁

重庆医科大学第一附属医院　血管外科

今年我承担"外科手术基础"这门课程的本科生教学，上课的地点是学校的图书馆。我突然意识到，这竟然是我到现在的工作单位任职超过十年以来，第一次走进学校的图书馆。

不过好像也没有那么奇怪，毕竟在我21世纪10年代的大学期间，除了因为一门叫"医学信息学"课程是在图书馆里上课之外，我也没有怎么去过图书馆。可那毕竟是中国医学科学院、北京协和医学院的图书馆啊！与病历、老教授一齐列在"协和三宝"的图书馆。

但又如何呢？

在互联网之前的时代，专业信息来源有限，图书馆里的学术期刊无疑是获取国外最新讯息最好的途径。而以期刊全面而著称的中国医学科学院北京协和医学院图书馆，在20世纪40年代，馆藏图书、期刊数即达到7万5千之多，400多种世界一流医学期刊从创刊号至今被完整收藏，这毫无疑问与协和在国内医学界首屈一指的地位相辅相成，也当之无愧地在"协和三宝"中拥有一席之地。据说当年在图书馆，可以不时地见到从外地乘坐各种交通工具赶到北京，专门到这里查询和查阅医学资料的学者。

但是，互联网已经解构了"图书馆"的神圣地位，甚至由于期刊数量的爆炸性增长，任何单一的图书馆都难以敢言"全面"。在新冠大流行期间，以跨越传统期刊同行评议周期的预出版模式为代表的新专业交流信息传播模式，又进一步改变了专业资讯获取渠道，也进一步侵蚀着传统图书馆的根基。图书馆，对于当代医学生来说，可能更多地变成了一个自习室，而不是查阅知识的场所。

想想也是，哪一种传统的形式不是在新时代不可阻挡地来临之际，被恋恋不舍地放弃的呢？那在这样的背景之下，图书馆，仍然配得上"协和三宝"吗？

不只是图书馆，病历、老教授，在北京协和医学院建立百年之后的今日，都不同程度地面临着挑战和冲击。

协和的医学界老教授，曾代表着协和在中国现代医学发展史上无可比拟的地位传奇。中华医学会成立的第一批12个专科学会创始会长中，有9人来自协和；1955年，中国科学院第一批学部委员中，来自协和的占医学界的三分之二；协和先后汇聚超过50名两院院士。老教授，是协和在中国医学领域一言九鼎的地位象征。

然而当下，医疗技术和理念的快速迭代，老教授的临床经验和观念变得不那么至关重要，信息化时代之下医学教育也已经不再依赖师承教授，那么老教授的价值到底如何体现呢？我觉得老教授的精神传承可能是不可替代的永远的瑰宝，他们对于医学的严谨求真的执着，对于病患认真负责的态度是一种宝贵精神遗产。

讲到病历、老协和，孙中山、宋庆龄、梁启超……大量名人病历见证并成就了协和在中国医学界历史上独特的传奇。同时协和留存着大量疑难病、罕见病病历，中国首例乃至世界首例病历，是世界范围内不可多得、难以复制的珍贵财富。

但是在信息化、无纸化的浪潮之下，伴随着医院规模扩大，平均住院时间缩短，周转率提升的时代背景，临床病历质量下降已经成为一个难以破解的现实问题，而这又动摇了病历价值的根基。

那么病历的价值到底是什么？

沉睡的文字，本身没有价值。病历是临床医疗、科研、教学最基础的原始素材，经归纳、整合、提炼、总结，最终汇聚成病历的临床价值。在我的学生时代，做一些临床科研是需要借病历的。进入病案科，站在巨大的病历档案库面前，那是"协和三宝"之一的"病历"给我最具象化的震撼。

而我的师弟师妹们不会再感受到这种震撼了，因为信息化时代已经不再需要从故纸堆里探寻。但是信息化不应该只是单纯实现电子化，而更应是对信息更为高效的整理。信息化运用的程度，决定了病历价值的高低。

试想，当你通过一个手术名称，可以看到系统统计的某个时间段内所有接受该种手术患者的基本信息分布、术中平均出血量、手术时长、术后并发症情况、平均住院时间等等，我相信那也是一种巨大的震撼，一种数字时代的震撼。

所以不是"协和三宝"是不是不再有意义的问题，而是在新的时代该如何去应用、发展的问题。

就像图书馆的信息系统如果能和病历系统进行某种对接整合，从被动等待被查阅的信息资源系统，变成主动推送的信息提供系统，又会对临床工作方式和流程带来怎样的颠覆？

同样，病历质量下降的问题，也可以通过信息化的手段来解决。结构化病历的初衷，就是以标准化提升临床工作效率的同时，也以标准化保证关键信息的完整性，同时又为后续的数据分析整合提供了基础。

写到这里时候，我会觉得，写病历甚至都不再需要医生去做，它已经变成了单纯的信息录入，甚至人工智能能干得更好。

但是，真是如此吗？我学生时代的经历，让我不免对我自己写的内容，产生了些许怀疑。记得一个西方医学教育名家说过：一切规则都是被用来打破的。

在内科实习时，我们被要求完成12份手写病历，并且我们每个学生，都被一对一地分配了一位老教授作为"病历导师"指导修改病例。我没有想到老教授这么认真。当我第一次诚惶诚恐地把病历交过去，她并没有当面批阅，而是说她先仔细看看，等她批阅完之后，再专门跟我约时间讲解。

"我感觉你好像不知道怎么写鉴别诊断"，在约定的讲解时间，病历导师跟我讲的第一句话颇让我意外，也让我困惑。鉴别诊断，难道不是这么写的？

"你的鉴别诊断是按照教科书来写的，书上说这个病要和哪些疾病进行鉴别，所以你就写要和什么疾病鉴别。但是没有患者会按照教科书的方式来生病啊？实际上，写鉴别诊断是反映我们在实际中的临床思维的，患者有些什么症状，有些什么体征，有哪些检查结果，这样的症状、体征和检查结果，可能提示什么样的疾病，有哪些症状、体征和检查结果是支持这个诊断的，又有哪些症状、体征和检查结果是不支持的？这才是真正的鉴别诊断。"

看着用红笔逐一细致标注修改的病历，听着病历导师耐心的讲解，那一刻我第一次认识到"协和三宝"中病历和老教授的意义。

病历，不只是病历本身，也是病历写作过程中对严谨、求实医学临床思维的训练过程，它是教学手段，也是这种教学模式下产生的成果。而老教授，不是简单指代学术权威，而是一代代协和大师对医学精益求精，对患者真心真情的精神力量，又通过教学，一代代薪火相传。

"协和三宝"，是具体的，更是抽象的。

它的载体，会随着时代变化而改变。就像我今年之所以会在图书馆里上课，是因为图书馆的部分楼层，被改造成了学校新的技能培训中心。

但"协和三宝"的精神内核，是永恒的。

就像如今当我查房的时候，有时候会很自然地握着患者的手，就像我的老师们曾经做过的那样。那是医学的温度，也是在协和医学教育中的温度。

于是，当我写下这些文字来探讨"协和三宝"时，探讨其实不应仅仅局限在去挖掘"协和三宝"的内涵意义，而应是怎么在新的时代背景下，如何去发挥"协和三宝"的价值？是否该有新时代下的新"协和三宝"？

这个讨论，也是关于北京协和医学院，这座曾经中国至高无上的医学殿堂，今天靠什么去实现自己的"区分度"，去标定自己在中国医学界甚至世界医学界的地位？

作为一个离开协和，现在就职在中国其他医学院校和教学医院的我，一方面觉得各个医学院校以及教学医院的提升，使得协和不再显得那么一枝独秀，对于中国医学教学未必不是一件幸事，毕竟14亿人口的大国，如果只有一个协和，其实反而是不正常的现象。另一方面，我又真诚地希望，协和能够再次引领中国医学以及医学教育在这个全新时代下探索发展，去续写协和的传奇。

"PUMC's Three Treasures" : can their glory remain?

Fu Qining

Department of Vascular Surgery, the First Affiliated Hospital of
Chongqing Medical University, Chongqing, China

Keywords: Medical education; PUMC's Three Treasures; medical record

This year, I took on the task of teaching the "Fundamentals of Surgery" course to undergraduate students in the school library. It dawned on me that this marked my first visit to the library in over a decade of working at my current institution.

To be honest, it's not surprising at all, given that during my university years in the 2010s, I rarely visited the library except for attending the "Medical Informatics" course held there. What truly amazed me was the fact that this library, where the course was held was none other than the library of the Chinese Academy of Medical Sciences and Peking Union Medical College (CAMS & PUMC)—a library held in the same high regard as the esteemed professors and medical records of Peking Union Medical College (PUMC), the three treasures of PUMC!

But what does this signify, after all?

Before the advent of the Internet, access to professional information was limited, and academic journals in the library undoubtedly served as the best way to stay updated with the latest international research. The library of the CAMS & PUMC, renowned for its extensive collection of journals, had amassed over 75,000 books and more than 400 world-class medical journals since the 1940s. This undoubtedly reflected PUMC's leading position in the Chinese medical field, earning the library a well-deserved place among the "Three Treasures of PUMC". It is said that back in the day, individuals from different regions of the country frequently traveled to Beijing solely to conduct research with medical information at the library.

However, the Internet has diminished the importance of libraries over time, and due to the exponential growth in the number of journals, it has become challenging for any single library to claim to have a truly "comprehensive" collection. During the COVID-19 pandemic, the new form of professional information dissemination called "pre-published", by passing the traditional peer-review process of journals, gained more attention and recognition. This further altered the means of accessing professional information and had a great impact on traditional libraries. For today's medical students, the library perhaps transitioned into more of a study space rather than a place for acquiring knowledge.

In fact, as the new era approaches, traditions are often reluctantly abandoned. Given this consideration, can the library still be regarded as one of the "Three Treasures of PUMC"?

A renowned medical education expert saying, *"All rules are meant to be broken."* Not only the library, but medical records and esteemed professors all encounter challenges to varying degrees after a century of PUMC's establishment.

The esteemed professors of PUMC once represented an unparalleled legend in the history of medical development in China. Nine out of the first twelve founding presidents of the Chinese Medical Association's specialty societies hailed from PUMC. In 1955, two-thirds of the medical members among the initial members of the Chinese Academy of Sciences were from PUMC. With over 50 academicians and esteemed professors gathered throughout the years, they epitomized PUMC's unquestionable standing in the Chinese medical field.

However, in light of the rapid advancements in medical technology and shifting ideologies, the clinical experience and perspectives offered by esteemed professors carry less weight in today's context, as medical education no longer relies exclusively on mentorship from professors. This raises the question of how we can truly acknowledge the value that esteemed professors bring.

Regarding medical records, the extensive collection of records of renowned individuals such as Sun Yat-sen, Soong Ching-ling, and Liang Qichao, among others, has played a crucial role in shaping the unique narrative of PUMC in the history of Chinese medicine. Furthermore, these records encompass numerous accounts documenting challenging and rare diseases, including notable instances of being the first case in China or even the world. These records constitute invaluable treasures that are both scarce and impossible to replicate on a global scale.

However, with the rise of information technology and the shift towards paperless records, along with the expansion of hospitals, shortened average length of hospital stays, and increased turnover rates, the declining quality of clinical medical records become a genuine concern, undermining the very foundation of the value of medical records.

So, what is the value of medical records?

Records that remain dormant hold no value. Medical records serve as the fundamental raw material for clinical medicine, scientific research, and education. Through summarization, integration, extraction, and synthesis, they embody the clinical value of records. During my student days, access to records was necessary for conducting clinical research. Standing before the vast archives of medical records in the Medical Records Department, one of the "Three Treasures of PUMC", left a lasting impact on me.

However, my younger colleagues will no longer experience such an impact, as information technology no longer requires delving into stacks of dated archives. Yet, information technology should not merely involve digitization but also provide efficient information organization. The extent to which information technology is utilized determines the value of medical records.

Imagine when you mention a surgical procedure, you can immediately retrieve a complete collection of basic information regarding all the patients who have undergone that surgery within a specific period. This collection would provide details like the average amount of bleeding during the operation, the duration of the surgery, any postoperative complications, and the average duration of hospitalization, etc. I firmly believe that such an advancement would be a remarkable breakthrough, exemplifying the power of the digital era.

Consequently, the question is not whether the "Three Treasures of PUMC" still hold significance but rather how to apply and develop them in this new era.

Similarly, the integration of the library's information system with the medical records system holds immense potential, transforming passive information resources into proactive providers. This integration can revolutionize clinical workflows and processes.

Likewise, information technology can address the issue of declining quality in medical records. The original intention of structured medical records is to standardize and improve clinical work efficiency while ensuring the integrity of key information and providing a foundation for subsequent data analysis and integration.

At this point, I can't help but feel that writing medical records no longer requires the presence of doctors. It seems to become a mere data entry task, or perhaps artificial intelligence could do it better.

However, is that truly the case? My experiences during my student days have made me doubt the content I wrote myself.

During my internal medicine rotation, we were required to complete twelve handwritten medical records, and each student was assigned a senior professor as a "medical record mentor" to guide and revise our writing. I didn't anticipate the mentor to take this assignment so seriously. When I nervously handed in my first writing records, she did not respond right away. Instead, she told me that she would carefully review it and then arrange a specific time to discuss its details with me.

"You need to work more on differential diagnosis", said my medical record mentor during our scheduled discussion. Her words surprised me and left me perplexed. Isn't that how a differential diagnosis is supposed to be written?

"You wrote the differential diagnosis based solely on what the textbooks state. The textbooks provide a list of diseases for consideration in the differential diagnosis, and you simply include those diseases for differentiation. However, patients don't get sick according to the textbook, do they? The process of writing the differential diagnosis involves reflecting on our clinical thinking based on the particular patient. What symptoms, signs, and test results does the patient exhibit? Based on these factors, what diseases might be indicated? And which symptoms, signs, and test results support or contradict this diagnosis? That's the true essence of a differential diagnosis."

As I observed the meticulous *red* markings on the record and listened to explanations from my mentor, I realized for the first time the significance of medical records and the role of esteemed professors in the "Three Treasures of PUMC".

Medical records go beyond mere documentation; they serve as a training process that nurtures rigorous and practical clinical thinking when writing. They act as teaching tools, and they represent the outcomes of this educational approach. Similarly, *the* term "professor" does not simply denote academic authority; it embodies the spirit of excellence in medicine and genuine care for patients that has been passed down through generations of PUMC professors through teaching. Their unwavering commitment to rigorous and genuine medical practice, coupled with their responsibilities in patient care, represents the enduring and irreplaceable spiritual legacy left behind by esteemed professors.

The "Three Treasures of PUMC" are concrete yet abstract. Their manifestation may change with time. For instance, this year I lecture in the library because a portion of the library was transformed into a new skills training center.

However, the spiritual core of the "Three Treasures of PUMC" remains. When I participate in ward rounds, sometimes I naturally hold the patient's hand, just as my teachers used to do, which represents the warmth of medicine as a part of PUMC's patient-centered spirit.

Therefore, as I pen these words to delve into the "Three Treasures of PUMC", the discussion should not be limited to uncovering their inherent meaning. It should also delve into how to find the value of the "Three Treasures of PUMC" in today's medical society and whether new "Three Treasures of PUMC" should be established.

This discussion is also about PUMC, once the supreme medical institution in China, how does it define its own uniqueness and establish its standing in the field of Chinese and even global medicine today?

As someone who has left PUMC and now works in a teaching hospital of another medical institution, I possess mixed perspectives. On one hand, I feel that the progress of various medical schools and teaching hospitals make PUMC no longer the sole outstanding institution. This is not a negative outcome for medical education in China. After all, in a country with a population of 1.4 billion, it would be abnormal to rely solely on one institution like PUMC. On the other hand, I sincerely hope that PUMC can once again lead Chinese medical education in this new era, continuing its legendary journey.

主编导读（二十二）

专家共识，能够更好指导临床工作吗？

我们需要什么样的专家共识？

我学医出道时，记忆中医学各个专业的指南和专家共识是不多的。如果有，老一辈专家也是非常慎重的，其内容和形式往往具有很高的权威性，对临床实践有明确的指导意义。

最近一些年来，医学各个学会的分支有了明显的增加和完善。不少"学会"的分支组织在中华医学会、中国医师协会和中国抗癌协会等主流学会之外，如雨后春笋般地生长。在有些没有太大关系的学会名下，也会挂上"肝胆外科分会"或者三级、四级分会。大家都能弄个话题，做一个平台，挺高兴。

与此相对应的是，各种"专家共识"被纷纷制定出来，名目繁多，而且还有不少重复，质量上当然不能完全顾及了。

但这也算是一个进步。因为年轻医生可以轻易查到本专业的专家共识，从中学到一些系统的、规范的内容，来指导他们的临床实践。因为现代社会再也不像早年一样，医生去读教科书或者翻阅纸版专业期刊了，专业知识的更新获得需要更加迅速和方便的途径。在这波"共识高潮"中，大部分制定的内容，虽然有重复、缺乏新意，但是至少在学术质量上还是比较靠谱的。

主要问题是这些纷纷出炉的共识制定过程参差不齐，文字和内容都让人有"行色匆匆""急于求成"的感觉。有些只是几位关系近的专家拉在一起，就制定一个共识，实际上只能算是几个专家的个别意见。上述这些共识很大一部分制定过程不够规范、严谨，往往是个别专家写一个比较完整的"大综述"（或者甚至让学生先写一个），找出一帮专家来提几个意见，修改后签上字，就完成了。

纵观西方发达国家制定的医学共识，就要严格得多，数量也少而精（虽然西方目前有集体打压我们的势头，但是他们有很多好的东西我们还是要学习，我们必须聪敏睿智到能把这两码事分开来对待）。制定一个正规的共识不仅花时间、精力，而且花费资金。单单开会、问答表格等流程就会有很多（如Delphi法，快速应用程序开发工具）。正规的共识需要的步骤包括：设置项目评估小组、编制专家咨询表、选择专家组（范围和人数都有规则）、开展三轮调查并对调查结果进行分析，然后对Delphi法研究结果进行统计，对专家意见的协调度和权威度进行评估，最后才形成一个专家共识。

只有这样严格规范操作，才能制定出一个有代表意义、具学术价值的专家共识。真正对临床医学起到较大的帮助作用。而我们目前看到的国内眼花缭乱的专家共识，一大部分都不是通过这种严格的方式制定出来的，其含金量自然会大打折扣。

在专家共识高潮过后，我们应该思考我们需要什么样的共识？需要多少专家共识？能不能代表中国学者的水平和工作风范？

就此问题我和上海复旦大学华山医院的陈进宏教授进行了交谈，他对此很有体会，并就此写了这篇文章。总体看，他对于我们的专家共识还是以正面看法为主。希望大家能就此发表各自的意见和看法。

专家共识——促进临床水平提升，最终使患者获益

陈进宏　　钦伦秀

复旦大学附属华山医院　普外肝胆外科中心

循证医学是现代医学的基石，基于目前的循证学证据，针对临床实际问题，由行业权威专家团队充分讨论，遵循规范流程，编写而成的专家共识可以为临床决策提供依据；另外，层出不穷的专家共识质量不尽一致，甚至有些观点不相符合，又给临床决策造成困惑。医学同道既盼望客观权威的专家共识指导临床工作，又时常感慨"这共识没啥用"。

目前有很多共识质量评估方法，例如AGREE Ⅱ（The Appraisal of Guidelines for Research and Evaluation，AGREE）、澳大利亚JBI循证卫生保健中心（2016）的真实性评价工具等；《中华医学杂志》也刊登《中国制定/修订临床诊疗指南的指导原则》（2022版），为提升专家共识质量提供指导，侧面也反映专家共识质量的良莠不齐。

笔者作为执笔者和专家组成员参与多部共识编写工作，日常工作中也通过学习专家共识，获益颇多。在此，个人想就编者和读者两个角度谈谈对共识的粗浅认识。

如何编写好共识

指南与共识的区分有时并不明确，普遍流行的观点是专家共识是一种质量和影响力低于指南的行业指导文件，指南参考的文献循证学证据级别更高，而专家共识强调专家经验在指南制定过程中发挥的作用，相关文献更多是探索性研究。

共识的选题

共识的选题应贴近临床，例如肝癌的转化治疗，虽说早有涉及，但近年来随着靶向免疫治疗的出现，肝癌转化治疗成为讨论热点，而相关的研究并不充分，通过颁布专家共识，可以及时给予规范性指导。

另一种是相关临床问题存在已久，但证据也不充分，如门静脉高压合并肝癌在国外往往被认为是外科手术禁忌证，而中国的临床实践手术相对积极，也积累了相当证据，针对这类问题制定共识，也有助于国内同道加深认识。

专家的组成

专家组成多为学术组织的专家团队，也有行业权威召集成立，优点是保证专家的权威性，但也可能导致意见偏差。

如同一学术组织的专家，由于平时交流多，意见会相对统一；而行业权威召集的专家，意见往往会偏向于召集人。

如果专家团队能包括一些其他领域的同行，共识意见可能会更客观，如制定手术相关共识，咨询一些内科以及介入科的专家，对手术指征的把握会谨慎一些；而制定腹腔镜手术的专家共识时，咨询一些平时不做腹腔镜手术的专家，对腹腔镜手术的优缺点的表述更为客观。

文献的全面解读

共识所谈论的问题基于参考文献的引证和分析，这就要求引用文献要全面，包含正反两方面观点的文献。

文献证据也不应直接转化成推荐意见，对于证据的解释需基于对文献进行充分分析、推理和论证的前提下，也应始终在患者的价值观和偏好的基础上加以考虑。

例如肝癌的系统治疗目前 A ＋ T（阿替利珠单抗联合贝伐珠单抗免疫联合疗法）的方案被美国国立综合癌症网络（NCCN）列为首

选，但考虑到国内患者的经济承受能力等，相关共识在推荐相关方案时也应充分考虑。

另外参加共识制定的专家大多在该领域作出了卓越贡献，共识一定也会引用到参与专家的研究工作成果。引用参与专家的文献时相对要更客观，如果是已被广泛认可的观点，引用无可厚非，但如果本身就是一家之言，在共识中展示就应该谨慎。

如果共识讨论问题为最新热点，相关研究更新速度就会很快，共识也应及时更新，以免读者接触到过时的信息。

制定过程的客观性

共识一般都是自发形成，但制定流程应该遵循透明性、规范性，以及推荐意见的独立性等客观标准。正式共识形成方法主要有4种，其中德尔菲法（Delphi Method）是最常用的一种。

最后观点的产生是"求同存异""少数服从多数"的结果，很难是所有专家一致同意的。

现在有些共识在观点争议较大时，会公布投票结果，甚至会咨询外部专家，这样对观点的产生有更客观的描述，更有利于读者客观理解。

如何读好共识

专家共识基于一定的文献支持，对临床问题高度总结，汇聚相关领域专家的集体智慧，是临床医生很好的学习途径。

学习共识是提高临床决策能力的要求

现在的医学是循证医学时代，随机对照研究作出来的荟萃分析站在证据金字塔的顶端，前瞻性随机/非随机对照研究和真实世界研究等均为临床问题提供很好的诊治依据，而个案报道和个人经验证据是最弱的。

现实中，相当数量的临床医生忙于日常工作，可能连中文文献都少有时间阅读，依赖的多是既往经验。

认真读好相关领域的专家共识，对于基层医院医生来说，有助于提高临床决策能力；从学习角度来说，也是事半功倍；对于大的医学中心医生来说，单中心的经验并不总是正确的，"兼听则明"，从专家共识中汲取不同经验，也是大有裨益。

共识并不限制临床决策选择

共识并非法规，而是推荐建议。如果临床工作完全遵循共识意见，医学也无从进步，患者也无法得到个体化精准治疗。

例如目前肝癌系统治疗方案的有效率在10%～30%，按照共识甚至指南推荐选择治疗方案，也意味着大部分患者接受的是无效治疗方案。

现在很多研究开始探索各种系统治疗方案的有效人群，由于证据尚不充分，共识很少采用。

临床医生处理患者时要结合临床实际、患者个体情况、医疗环境等综合判断，进行临床决策。

当有多个共识意见不同，甚至完全相左时，例如围绕着胆囊结石的"切"与"保"的问题，近年来就有意见截然不同的专家共识，这就需要临床医生深入学习相关文献，结合实际情况来判断相关意见的科学性和可行性。

由于不同国家或地区间文化、经济的差异，不同人种对于治疗疗效的差异，在参考国外指南或共识时，应结合国情酌情采用。

共识是临床研究课题的重要来源

临床研究有助于改进临床实践，临床医生也应积极开展临床研究，但如何选题往往成为难点。共识虽然一定程度上规范了临床工作，但同时很多意见的证据来源为观察性研究，而少有随机对照试验研究。

深入学习和理解共识，从中发现有意义的争议性问题，就是很好的临床研究方向。高级别的临床研究结果，反过来也促进共识质量的提高，临床医生也从证据使用者转变成证据提供者。

总结

总之，写好专家共识，读好专家共识，采用批判的态度和科学的方法对其进行解读，并选择性应用，促进临床水平提升，最终使患者获益。

参考文献

[1] Brouwers MC, Kho ME, Browman GP, et al. AGREE II: advancing guideline development, reporting and evaluation in health care. CMAJ 2010; 182: E839-42.

[2] Joanna Briggs Institute. The Joanna Briggs Institute Reviewers' Manual: 2016 edition. Australia: The Joanna Briggs Institute; 2016.

[3] Chen Y, Yang K, Wang X, et al. Guiding Principles for the Formulation/Revision of Clinical Diagnosis and Treatment Guidelines in China (2022 edition). Chinese Medical Journal 2022; 102: 697-703.

Expert consensus—promoting clinical excellence and ultimately benefitting patients

Chen Jinhong, Qin Lunxiu

Hepatobiliary Surgery, Department of General Surgery, Huashan Hospital, Fudan University, Shanghai, China

Keywords: Consensus; guideline; evidence-based medicine

Evidence-based medicine serves as the cornerstone of modern healthcare. Based on current evidence in the field of evidence-based medicine, a team of authoritative experts in the industry engages in comprehensive discussions to develop expert consensus, following standardized procedures. The consensus serves as a foundation for clinical decision-making. However, the abundance of expert consensus varies in quality, and some viewpoints even contradict each other, leading to confusion in clinical decision-making. Medical professionals expect authoritative expert consensus to guide their clinical work but, at times, express frustration, saying that the consensus is "useless". Various methods are currently available to assess the quality of consensus, such as AGREE II (The Appraisal of Guidelines for Research and Evaluation II) [1] and the credibility assessment tool from the Australian JBI Center for Evidence-Based Healthcare [2016] [2]. Additionally, "Guiding Principles for the Formulation/Revision of Clinical Diagnosis and Treatment Guidelines in China (2022 edition)" is published in the *Chinese Journal of Medicine* [3]. The emergence of numerous assessment tools stems from the dire need to evaluate and improve current expert consensus, reflecting the inconsistent quality of those consensus.

I have been a writer and a member of expert consensus groups participating in multiple consensus development projects. And the literature can often supply a decent amount of food for thought. As an author and reader, I would like to share some personal understanding of expert consensus from both perspectives.

Q1: How to write a good consensus?

The distinction between guidelines and consensus is not always clear, but it is generally believed that expert consensus is an industry guidance document with lesser influence and lower quality compared to guidelines. Guidelines refer to higher levels of evidence-based medicine, while expert consensus emphasizes the role of expert experience in the process of guideline formulation, relying more on exploratory research literature.

Topic selection for consensus

Consensus topics should be closely related to clinical practice. For instance, there have been, discussions on conversion therapy for liver cancer for a long time, but the emergence of targeted therapy and immunotherapy in recent years has truly made conversion therapy a hot topic. However, there might not be sufficient related research. By issuing expert consensus, timely standardized guidance can be provided for these new therapies. Another situation is when a clinical problem was discovered for a long time, but the evidence is still insufficient. For example, portal hypertension combined with liver cancer is often considered a surgical contraindication in many countries, while such clinical practices in China are relatively proactive and have gained considerable evidence. Developing consensus on such diseases can help Chinese doctors deepen their understanding.

Composition of expert panels

Expert panels are typically composed of experts from academic organizations or assembled by industry authorities. This approach ensures the expertise of panel members, but it may also lead to potential biases in their opinions. Experts from the same academic organization tend to share similar opinions due to frequent communication; experts convened by industry authorities, on the other hand, might tend to align with the convener's opinions. To enhance the objectivity of the consensus, it would be beneficial to include peers from other fields within the expert team. For example, when formulating consensus on surgical indications, consulting experts from internal medicine and interventional medicine can lead to more cautious considerations. Similarly, when formulating a consensus on laparoscopic surgery, consulting experts who do not typically perform such procedures can provide a more impartial assessment of its advantages and disadvantages.

Interpretation of literature

The context of consensus is analyzed and cited from clinical literature. This requires including comprehensive literature that presents both supportive and opposing viewpoints. The evidence from the literature should not be duplicated directly into recommendations. Instead, forming a consensus based on the evidence relies on thorough analysis and reasoning. Furthermore, patients' values and preferences should always be taken into account. For instance, the A+T regimen is currently listed as the first-line regimen for systemic treatment of liver cancer by National Comprehensive Cancer Network (NCCN). However, the economic background of certain patients should be thoroughly considered when recommending this regimen. Many experts contributing to the consensus have made significant impacts on the field, and the consensus will inevitably cite their research work. A relatively objective approach should be taken when this scenario happens. If the expert's viewpoint is widely recognized, citing it is justifiable; however, if the viewpoint represents a singular opinion, caution should be exercised when including it in the consensus. When the consensus addresses cutting-edge issues, it is important to promptly update the relevant research and consensus to ensure that readers are not exposed to outdated information.

Objectivity during the process

Consensus is generally naturally formed, but its formation process should follow objective standards such as transparency, normative, and independence of recommendations. There are primarily four formal methods for forming a consensus, with the Delphi Method being the most commonly used. The final consensus reflects the viewpoints of the majority, as per the principle of seeking common ground while reserving differences. Achieving a unanimous agreement among all experts is challenging if not impractical. Some recent consensus disclose the poll distribution when the conclusion is controversial. External experts may also be involved in the procedure. This provides a more objective description of how the viewpoints are formulated and allows the readers to perceive the viewpoints in an objective fashion.

Q2: How to read a consensus?

Expert consensus is a condensed overview of clinical problems supported by relevant literature, drawing upon the collective wisdom of experts in the field and offering a valuable learning pathway for clinical practitioners.

Learning from consensus to enhance clinical decision-making

Contemporary medicine follows evidence-based practices. At the

守在生命的边缘
医者沉思录

apex of the evidence pyramid are meta-analyses of randomized controlled trials. Prospective randomized/non-randomized controlled studies, along with real-world research, establish robust foundations for clinical problem-solving. Conversely, case reports and personal empirical evidence hold the lowest evidentiary value. In practice, many clinicians are occupied with their daily duties, leaving them little time for extensive literature review, often relying predominantly on their past clinical experiences. For local clinic physicians, learning from consensus proves advantageous in refining their clinical decision-making, ultimately enhancing their clinical skills and yielding better outcomes with minimal effort. For physicians in major medical centers, experiences from a single institution may not be universally applicable; hence, gleaning insights from a range of perspectives within expert consensus can be beneficial.

Consensus does not limit clinical decisions

Consensus isn't a legal mandate but rather a set of recommended suggestions. Strictly adhering to consensus in clinical practice would impede treatment progress and hinder individualized treatment for patients. For instance, current systemic treatment regimens for liver cancer demonstrate efficacy rates of approximately 10% to 30%. Strictly following consensus or guidelines might lead to most patients receiving ineffective treatments. Many studies are now beginning to explore the effective population of various systemic treatment options, but due to insufficient evidence, consensus is rarely adopted. Clinical practitioners must consider reality factors including individual patient conditions and the medical environment to make informed clinical decisions. When confronted with multiple consensus opinions, particularly when opinions are opposed, as seen in the recent expert consensus on "resection" versus "preservation" regarding gallstones, clinicians should thoroughly examine relevant literature, assessing the scientific validity and feasibility of these opinions within the given context. Moreover, considering the cultural, economic, and ethnic variations across different countries or regions, contextual factors should be taken into account when referencing international guidelines or consensus.

Consensus as a valuable source for clinical research

Clinical research enhances clinical practices, and clinicians should actively engage in clinical research. However, topic selection often poses a challenge. While consensus provides some level of standardization in clinical work, many opinions rely on observational studies and lack randomized controlled trials. An in-depth understanding of consensus helps identify meaningful and contentious topics, creating excellent directions for clinical research. In return, the outcomes of high-level clinical research improve consensus quality, enabling clinicians to shift from being evidence learners to evidence contributors.

In summary, medical professionals should learn to interpret and write sound expert consensus, employ clinical and scientific methodologies, and apply it selectively in clinical work to improve decision-making and ultimately benefit patients.

References

[1] Brouwers MC, Kho ME, Browman GP, et al. AGREE II: advancing guideline development, reporting and evaluation in health care. CMAJ 2010; 182: E839-42.

[2] Joanna Briggs Institute. The Joanna Briggs Institute Reviewers' Manual: 2016 edition. Australia: The Joanna Briggs Institute; 2016.

[3] Chen Y, Yang K, Wang X, et al. Guiding Principles for the Formulation/Revision of Clinical Diagnosis and Treatment Guidelines in China (2022 edition). Chinese Medical Journal 2022; 102: 697-703.

主编导读（二十三）

中国基层医院的现状、困境和出路

中国的基层医疗走向何处？

仅仅数十年以前，我国普通民众的医疗保障水平还相当低下，可能主要顾及的还是吃饱饭、活下去、不在乱世中丢失性命。就像在有人抱怨为什么中国不早点、长期地投入基础研究时，我的一个朋友提出灵魂拷问：中国人作为整体，吃饱饭有多少年？

在改革开放以后，我国全民的医疗保障水平有了提高。医疗保障的机制和规则一直在摸索和修改中，实话说，和西方发达国家差距还是明显的。到底人均GDP摆在那里，这是不言而喻的。

我国一直有三级医疗体系，而且已经实施了一段时间。要照顾全世界最大数量的患者群体不是一件容易的事情。社会贫富不均、地区差异巨大是明显的问题。虽然整个医疗体系，尤其是基层医疗尚未完全理顺，而且一直在理，但不可否认进步还是明显的。因为整个经济情况、社会文明和社会秩序一直随着发展而改变，所以三级医疗体系、基层医院的走向等都在不断的调整中，还应该没有定式。目前大家都基本认同我们中国有中国的特殊国情，完全照搬西方现成的模式是不合适的。

我最近有机会去一个基层的县级医院会诊，发现作为中国医疗系统基本"细胞"的县医院还多少处于一种迷茫的困境之中。有关是不是要把县医院逐渐升级为大而全的三甲医院？有没有条件这么做？这么做是不是真的对全民医疗带来好处？这些问题还没有明确答案；有些地区要求县医院要把"大部分患者留在当地治疗"，这个是不是合理？能不能办到？对患者是不是真的好？莫衷一是。这些还是方向性问题，现存的问题还有县级医院如何保证财政，如何留住医科大学毕业的人才，是不是需要及如何开展高难度的手术等治疗等，都是在摸索中的事情。

总体来看，中国在目前国力下，所花费的资金，能够基本照顾好这么多的患者已经不容易。因为实际上发达国家对于医保体系也是焦头烂额、捉襟见肘。希望这些现有的问题能够随着国力的增强、经济的进一步发展，慢慢消化掉。回顾改革开放初期，也曾经有很多看上去没法解决的难题，无法逾越的障碍，随着经济的发展和社会的进步，自然而然显得不那么要命了，有些还得到了解决。希望医疗体系也会是这样把问题解决了。所以对于国家，做好自己的事情，使得经济持续发展才是硬道理。

就中国基层医院的现状、困境和出路，最有发言权的还是基层医院的领导，在此我邀请了我多年的老朋友——辽宁省开原市中心医院（县级医院）的张戈院长来写这篇文章，他在这家医院里担任科主任和院领导多年，经历了很多变迁，请他来讲讲他所经历的第一手材料。

中国基层医院的现状、困境和出路

王子怡[1]　张　戈[2]

[1]辽宁省中医药大学
[2]辽宁省开原市中心医院

同世界各国的基层医疗服务比较，中国现有的基层医疗体系有其特殊性。这同我国的现行体制、国情和民族传统有一定的关系，也同急速发展和急剧变化的经济、医疗保障系统有关。同其他很多领域一样，与其说是到了一个成熟、相对稳定的阶段，不如说一直是走在一条不断探索、改善、进步的路上。出现问题和不尽完善是不令人惊讶的。毕竟，中国人全体脱贫才多少年。

人类社会从进化以来，还从没有经历过占本种族近五分之一的人口集体脱贫，且集体需要医疗保障的过程。基层医疗要过河，连摸的石头都没有。

中国基层医院的现状

和西方发达国家业已存在多年并相对行之有效的基层医疗体制不一样，目前我国基层医疗尚需完善与加强。其中以县级公立医院为龙头，引领乡医院、村医组成基层三级医疗网，而作为龙头的县级医院承载与上级医院相连接的功能，起到了承上启下的作用，在基层医疗体系中县医院成为重中之重。

2012年以来，县级公立医院的医疗改革一直在推进中，试图提升县级医院的能力，其中有"破除以药养医为切入点的县级公立医院综合改革""县级医院医疗服务能力提升工程""五个中心建设""医联体及医共体的建设"等多项政策。这些医疗改革措施的本意是提高县医院的综合服务能力，实现90%患者留在县域，大病不出县。

事实上，通过一些政策的扶持，部分县医院的整体服务能力得到了明显提升，有的县医院已经进入三级医院行列，甚至三甲医院。但是有些措施的效果明显没有达到设计初衷。尤其是经济欠发达地区，有相当一部分县级医院仍然存在很多困难，财力不足、人才奇缺、科室建设和发展缓慢，重大疾病的救治能力不足，造成患者流失比较严重，实现"大病不出县"的目标之路还很漫长，或者永远达不到。

基层医疗的困境

财力不足

县级医院是差额拨款事业单位，除了自营收入外，经营缺口需要县级财政补充。但欠发达地区的财政刚性都难以自保，对医院的投入微乎其微。本应由政府解决的建设、设备、仪器购置及人才培养等所需资金问题全部转到医院上来，使医院举步维艰。

医院在维持人员正常开资的前提下，只能通过贷款融资等途径来解决上述问题。虽解一时之急，但也给医院增加了额外的负担，出现了负债经营，大部分医院负债率达百分之五十以上，有的甚至超百分之百。

医疗人才的流失

财力不足也直接影响了人才培养和引进，目前县级医院招录的毕业生以本科生为主，新的毕业生面临两个考试，一个是执业医师考试，一个是专业医生规范化培训，基本需要4～5年时间，这期间他们一直忙于培训或考试，医院要承担其培训费用却不能派遣临床工作，当他们通过考试或培训取得证书后，就有了到更高层次医院聘任的资格。由于基层医院工资待遇偏低，学科建设不完善，有相当一部分新人拿到证书后辞职去往上级医院或经济发达地区，仅有少部分原籍或周边城镇的人留下来，近十年新生流失比例在60%以上，造成了新人补充严重不足。

而医院原来一些有能力的医生也在向经济发达地区流动；民营医院还在高薪挖人，还有一些专家也到了退休年龄，几个方面原因造成人才匮乏。医生忙于日常临床工作，医院也很少能抽出人员去上级医院进修学习，也制约了学科的建设与发展。

学科建设缓慢

县级医院为实现"大病不出县"的目标，都在向更高的级别医院（三级或三甲）晋升而努力，就必然开展新的学科及各种中心建设，但学科建设也离不开资金投入及相关人才的培养。为开展新的学科，医院宁可负债也要购置昂贵的大型设备，但人才问题不是短期内能解决的，这样就出现了新设备的操作及诊断都不是短期内能达到很高水平的现象，项目开展受到限制。

以胸痛中心、卒中中心为例，设备安装后往往缺少专业操作人员及医生，难以形成团队，需要和上级医院的医生联合，由他们临时来帮助操作解决诊疗问题，这就有一个时间窗的问题，加之本院人员和外来专家的配合需要有一个熟悉过程。这些常常使得诊治患者的预后达不到最佳结果，患者接受度也不高；设备使用率低下，形成另一种浪费。学科建设速度缓慢也就是必然。结果是有的医院级别上去了，但业务能力和医疗水平与医院的级别并不完全匹配。

由于上面种种原因，必然出现患者向外流失的情况。另一方面医疗改革后出台了大量的惠民政策，方便百姓外地就医，让他们有了更多的选择。有些常见病、多发病，基层医院完全有能力解决，但患者也宁可去大医院治疗，而大医院也乐意收治，这也是县域患者外流的原因。

县级医院为留住患者勉强开展一些大的手术及高新技术，但因本级医院人员能力所限及患者认知度不高，即便几经努力，一年下来也只能开展几例到十几例，数量很少，与实际需要不匹配。虽然方便了患者，也节省了他们的医疗费用，但这些大手术及高新技术开展过程中的规范性难以保证。愈后转归、合并症的控制问题显然与大医院不能相比。也有的医院尝试通过医疗联合体的形式与大医院联合来解决这个问题，但实践证明并不成功，因为上级医院很难投入大量的精力和人员，也很难覆盖全部基层医院，不能寄希望于此。

基层医疗改革的迷思

中国的县级医院都朝着三级医院升级的目标对不对，能不能实现？如果全国连基层医院都朝大而全的方向努力，那么基层医疗就不再"基层"了。同时晋级的县级"三甲医院"是否真有实力、人才和水平同大型三甲医院去比拼？

三甲医院是不是应该做基层医院能够完成的简单、初级手术，造成患者分配不均衡？

其实分级诊疗已经为我们指出了方向，但各级医院职能定位比较模糊，病种的收治也无规定可以遵循。患者去哪级医院就医基本由自己决定，虽有医保报销比例的不同作约束，但其实是顺其自然，分级诊疗难以落到实处。

大型三甲医院如何同基层医院合作？是否可以分类收治患者？针对大手术、重大内科疾病的患者，大型三甲医院和基层医院在整个治疗过程中可否合作和分段进行？如患者术后恢复、支持过程在基层医院进行，患者随访工作在基层医院进行。

从这方面看，留住90%的患者在县域，大病不出县是否合理？是否最后留得住？

基层医疗的出路

实话说，谁也不知道中国基层医疗改革的具体出路在哪儿，但是最终目标是明确的，就是我们最终要建立一个适合中国人的基层医疗服务系统，在这个系统里面，民众得到良好的照顾，社会体现出足够的温暖，前沿医疗、医学研究的探索得到充分的发挥。

有些大型三甲医院能够在先进医学领域里逐渐和世界接轨甚至部分超越，而民众的基本医疗需要又能够方便快速地得到照顾。一套完善的系统应该是各司其职、各自担当起不同的角色。我们完全有信心期待。

Primary hospitals in China: current state, challenges, and solutions

Wang Ziyi[1], Zhang Ge[2]

[1] Liaoning University of Traditional Chinese Medicine, Shenyang, China

[2] Kaiyuan Central Hospital of Liaoning Province, Kaiyuan, China

Keywords: Primary hospitals; primary healthcare services; healthcare systems; healthcare reform

When it comes to primary healthcare services, China's primary medical system stands out with its unique attributes, shaped by China's existing framework, cultural heritage, and the rapid growth of its economy and healthcare sector. Unlike established systems in the West, the healthcare landscape of China is in a constant state of evolution, adapting to its ever-changing society. It's no surprise that challenges abound, especially given that it's been only a few decades since nearly one-fifth of the Chinese population collectively lifted themselves out of poverty and required access to healthcare coverage. Navigating the complexities of primary healthcare in China feels akin to crossing a river blindly, stepping on stones people can't see.

The current state of primary hospitals in China

In contrast to the robust healthcare systems in developed Western nations, China's primary healthcare system still requires significant improvements. Among them, county-level public hospitals serve as the leading constitutions that connect with higher-level hospitals, leading township hospitals and village clinics to form a three-tiered primary healthcare network. Since 2012, county-level public hospitals have undergone continuous reforms, striving to improve their capabilities. Various initiatives like "Comprehensive Reform of County-level Public Hospitals on Breaking the Pharmaceutical-Driven Model", "Capacity Improvement Project for County Hospitals", "Establishment of Five Centers", and "Development of Medical Alliances and Medical Communities" have been introduced. The goal behind these reforms is to bolster the service capabilities of county hospitals, ensuring that 90% of patients can receive proper treatment within their own counties, even for complicated diseases.

While these policies have undoubtedly bolstered several county hospitals, transforming them into tertiary institutions, some measures have fallen short. Particularly in economically disadvantaged regions, county hospitals grapple with financial constraints, a dearth of skilled professionals, sluggish departmental growth, and limited capacity to treat major diseases. Consequently, a considerable number of patients seek healthcare elsewhere. Achieving the objective of providing comprehensive local treatment for major diseases remains an arduous and prolonged journey or may never be achieved.

Challenges in primary healthcare

Inadequate funding

County-level hospitals rely on varying government subsidies. Apart from self-operated income, these hospitals need financial aid from county governments to bridge the operational gap. However, financially disadvantaged regions struggle to allocate ample funds, burdening these hospitals. Responsibilities such as infrastructure, equipment procurement, and personnel training, typically government-led, are transferred to hospitals, intensifying their challenges. To cope with regular expenses, hospitals resort to loans, creating additional financial strains. Many hospitals operate under significant debt, with debt ratios exceeding 50% and sometimes reaching 100%.

Loss of healthcare professionals

Insufficient funding directly affects the recruitment and training of healthcare professionals. County-level hospitals mainly recruit doctors with undergraduate degrees. These young doctors face two exams: the medical practitioner exam and specialized physician standardized training, a process lasting 4 to 5 years. During this period, hospitals bear training costs with little clinical contributions. Due to low salaries and limited specialism development of primary hospitals, many graduates leave for higher-tier hospitals or prosperous regions after certification. Over the last decade, the trained healthcare employees' outflow rate exceeded 60%. Skilled doctors also migrate to economically developed regions, attracted by lucrative offers from private hospitals. This, coupled with retirements, contributes to a scarcity of healthcare personnel in county-level hospitals. Daily clinical duties make it hard for hospitals to send staff for advanced training, further hindering medical discipline growth.

Slow progress in discipline development

To achieve the goal of providing comprehensive local healthcare, primary healthcare centers are striving to upgrade to higher-tier or tertiary hospitals. This necessitates the establishment of new disciplines and various centers. Discipline development requires substantial financial investment and the recruitment of relevant professional staff. Hospitals are willing to incur debts to purchase expensive large-scale equipment for new disciplines. However, professional training is a long-term endeavor. Consequently, the operation and diagnosis using new equipment cannot reach a high level immediately, limiting project implementation. For instance, in centers for chest pain or stroke, a lack of specialized operators and doctors often persists after equipment installation. This necessitates temporary collaboration with doctors from higher-tier hospitals to assist in operations and address diagnostic challenges. This interim arrangement, coupled with the need for synergy between hospital staff and external experts, often leads to suboptimal patient outcomes and low patient satisfaction. The underutilization of equipment results in inefficiencies. The slow pace of discipline development is inevitable. Consequently, although some hospitals have elevated their levels, their operational capacity and medical standards do not fully align with their hospital levels.

Due to these challenges, patients tend to seek healthcare elsewhere. Additionally, after the healthcare reformation, several policies were issued to facilitate medical treatment in non-local areas, providing patients with more options. In fact, despite the ability of primary healthcare centers to handle common diseases, patients prefer seeking treatment in large hospitals. Large hospitals readily admit patients, leading to the outflow of patients from primary healthcare centers.

To retain patients, primary healthcare centers attempt to perform a number of major surgeries and high-tech procedures. However, due to limited staff capabilities and disease awareness, their efforts fall short of the actual need. Although these attempts are convenient for patients and reduce their medical expenses, ensuring the quality of major surgeries and high-tech procedures remains a challenge. Postoperative outcomes and complications are not comparable to those in large hospitals. Some hospitals attempt to address this by forming alliances with larger institutions. However, this approach has shown limited success, as higher-tier hospitals struggle to invest significant resources and staff across all primary healthcare centers. A solution in this direction appears increasingly unlikely.

Thoughts about primary healthcare reform

Is every county-level hospital in China truly progressing toward the goal of becoming a tertiary institution? Is this feasible? If all primary healthcare centers in the nation aspire to be comprehensive, the essence of primary healthcare would lose its fundamental nature. Furthermore, do the county-level "tertiary hospitals" possess the expertise and service to compete with large tertiary A hospitals?

Should tertiary A hospitals perform basic surgeries that primary healthcare centers can manage, causing an unbalanced distribution of patients?

The tiered healthcare policy points out the direction for us. However, the functional roles of hospitals at different tiers remain unclear, and there are no specific guidelines for admitting different types of diseases. Patients largely decide which hospital level to visit, despite certain restrictions based on various medical insurance reimbursement rates. Implementing the tiered healthcare policy effectively is difficult.

How can large tertiary A hospitals collaborate with primary healthcare centers? Can patients be categorized for treatment? Can patients be carried out in stages for major surgeries and chronic diseases throughout the entire treatment process? For example, post-operative recovery and supportive treatment could occur at primary healthcare centers, and patient follow-ups as well.

From this standpoint, is it reasonable to solve 90% of patients' healthcare needs within the county, ensuring major diseases are not referred to outside the county? Can this goal be realistically achieved?

The future of primary healthcare

To be honest, the specific path for reforming primary healthcare in China remains uncertain. However, the ultimate objective is clear: to establish a primary healthcare service system tailored for the Chinese people, that is, the public receives excellent care, and cutting-edge medical exploration and research are fully utilized. Certain large tertiary A hospitals are gradually aligning with global standards in advanced medical fields, with some even surpassing these standards. Meanwhile, the fundamental healthcare needs of the public should be met conveniently and swiftly. Each component within the system should have well-defined roles and responsibilities. We are confident in anticipating this prospect.